CHALLENGES IN PUBLIC HEALTH GOVERNANCE:
THE CANADIAN EXPERIENCE

CLAUDE M. ROCAN

CHALLENGES IN PUBLIC HEALTH GOVERNANCE:
THE CANADIAN EXPERIENCE

CLAUDE M. ROCAN

INVENIRE BOOKS
Ottawa, Canada
2012

© INVENIRE BOOKS 2012

Library and Archives Canada Cataloguing in Publication

Rocan, Claude
    Challenges in public health governance: the Canadian
experience / Claude M. Rocan

Includes bibliographical references.
Issued also in electronic format.
ISBN 978-0-9877575-8-6 (print format)

        1. Public health administration--Canada.
2. Medical policy--Canada. I. Title.

RA449.R639 2012   362.10971   C2012-903780-X

Invenire Books would like to gratefully acknowledge the financial support
for the publication of this book by the Centre on Governance, University
of Ottawa.

Published by Invenire
P.O. Box 87001
Ottawa, Canada K2P 1X0
www.invenire.ca

Cover design by Sandy Lynch
Cover image by Wuka | Dreamstime.com
Layout and design by Sandy Lynch

Printed in Canada by Marquis Imprimeur Inc.

Distributed by:
Commoners' Publishing
631 Tubman Cr.
Ottawa, Canada K1V 8L6
Tel.: 613-523-2444
Fax: 613-260-0401
sales@commonerspublishing.com
www.commonerspublishing.com

TABLE OF CONTENTS

I – SETTING THE STAGE

II – PUBLIC HEALTH GOVERNANCE IN CANADA: THREE THEATRES

CHAPTER 7 – GLOBAL DRIVERS

IV – DEVELOPING THE TOOLS

CHAPTER 8 – FACING THE TOUGH QUESTIONS

CHAPTER 9 – TOWARDS A NETWORK GOVERNANCE REGIME IN PUBLIC HEALTH

To my wife, Anna,
and my parents,
Maurice and Jeanne

PREFACE

So why a book on network governance and public health in Canada? Why is this important for Canada and why is it important for public health?

I can think of several reasons:

1. Public health is important for the health and well-being of Canadians. Indeed, in spite of receiving only two to three percent of the health care system budget, public health may have contributed as much or more to the improvements in health that we have seen over the past century as has the health care system. A case in point is the quite dramatic decline in cardiovascular disease mortality in the past 30 years; the evidence suggests that this decline is due in roughly equal measure to prevention (the realm of public health and clinical prevention) and improved treatment. Another equally dramatic emerging trend is the decline in lung cancer mortality in men (women are a decade or two behind), which is due almost entirely to prevention, and not due to improved treatment; the prognosis from diagnosis has not markedly changed in recent decades.

   Another way that public health is important to Canadians, and perhaps one that comes more immediately to the minds of the public, is its role in preventing and combatting outbreaks of infectious disease. Indeed, as Claude notes, it was the SARS outbreak, coming on the heels of the outbreak of E. coli, linked to contaminated drinking in Walkerton, Ontario, and several other very public episodes, that led to the creation of the Public Health Agency of Canada and the Pan-Canadian Public Health Network. Canadians and their political leaders

CHALLENGES IN PUBLIC HEALTH GOVERNANCE

(finally) became aware of the neglect that public health had suffered, and demanded improvements.

It is ironic, then, that public health and prevention, in general, are not included within the *Canada Health Act*. The result: the federal government does not contribute to the funding of public health in Canada in the way it contributes to diagnosis, treatment and care. That situation no doubt exacerbates the neglect that public health suffers.

It is important, by the way, to be clear about what is meant by 'public health'. There has been an unfortunate tendency in recent years among political leaders and the 'chattering classes' to talk about 'public health care' when they mean publicly funded health care, otherwise (and equally incorrectly) known as Medicare (which is an American program). Public health is a long-established government service within society, focused on improving the health of the population and reducing inequalities in health through health promotion, health protection and disease prevention. It traces its roots to the mid-19th century, and thus predates publicly-funded health care by roughly a century in Canada.

2. Public health problems are often good examples of 'wicked problems' – complex, multi-factorial, often long-term, requiring a wide variety of interventions, and beset with multiple stakeholders, conflicts between public benefit and private profit, and between collective and individual rights. Understanding how to address and manage such wicked problems in public health may have lessons for how to address them in areas such as climate and ecological change, poverty and social equity, and the like.

3. Like it or not (and increasingly, I am not sure I do), we live in a federation, with a marked separation of powers between the federal and provincial governments, especially in the area of health. Constitutionally, health is a provincial responsibility, and maybe that works for the provision of treatment services, although even here there are problems. But typically, public health problems don't respect human-created boundaries; this is most obviously true for infectious diseases, but smoking, fast foods, environmental pollutants, urban sprawl and poverty, to name just a few current major public health problems, are global in scope.

So our governments need to find ways to effectively work together across Canada and, indeed, internationally if we are to fulfill the mission of public health. Learning the strengths and weaknesses of network governance, and how and when to apply it, is thus of great importance.

4. Governance is more than government, a point made memorably (for me) by Osborne and Gaebler in their 1991 book, *Reinventing Government*. They stated: "Governance is the process by which we collectively solve our problems and meet our society's needs. Government is the instrument we use." While I would argue that government is not *the* instrument we use, but one of the instruments – perhaps the main instrument – their point is very important. A collective process of solving problems and meeting needs, whether at the local level or at the global level, will involve many sectors across the community or society – public, private, non-profit, academic, faith, community – as well as individuals. So clearly, the ability to apply network governance will be needed to manage this process of community and societal governance.

This issue is particularly important for public health work, especially work in the area known as population health, which is concerned with addressing the main determinants of health that largely lie beyond (and upstream of) the scope of the health care system. Improving the health of the population requires us to influence such important factors as food supply and quality, urban form, transportation systems, poverty reduction, alcohol marketing, housing design, policing and so on. While some, perhaps much of this can be handled through public policy, some cannot.

To take but one simple example, it seems unlikely that portion size in restaurants will be regulated by the government any time soon; portion size is, in essence – and will likely remain – a private policy. Yet the dramatic increase in portion size over the past few decades has been identified as one of the factors contributing to obesity, which is one of the major public health challenges we face. So how do we get what I call healthy private policy? If we are not going to regulate it – if we are not going to use what W.T. Stanbury referred to as the legitimate coercive power of a democratically elected government – then we have to use persuasion, we have to sit down with and, in some sense, become partners with the food industry.

In fact, that line of thinking is what lies behind the establishment of food policy councils, of which Toronto's is the oldest in Canada. While established and supported by Toronto City Council (in 1989), it is not mainly an instrument of public policy, but of community governance. Here farmers, food companies, restaurants, environmentalists, food banks, nutritionists, concerned citizens, public health staff and others work together to create a community food system that is good for health, the community, the environment and the economy. This is governance in action, although sadly, only at the municipal level; there are no food policy councils (or healthy housing policy councils, or healthy transportation policy councils – the list goes on) at the provincial or federal levels, although the occasional example of something like this can be found, such as the Healthy Child Manitoba Committee.

Central to this concept of governance for health is the need to recognize and accept the importance of partners beyond government. So it is unfortunate, to say the least, that the Public Health Network has in effect ejected its non-governmental partners from the expert group level (now represented by the new steering committees) and relegated them to the working group level, which is neither as influential nor permanent in nature. In my view this is a step back from good governance for public health.

In this book, Claude explores these and other issues both directly and indirectly through the lens of the Public Health Network (PHN). (Here I should point out that Claude and I worked together for several years as the first co-chairs of the Population Health Promotion Expert Group of the Pan-Canadian Public Health Network, he as the federal co-chair, me as the provincial/territorial co-chair; at that time, I worked as a population and public health consultant for the BC Ministry of Health).

The picture he paints is not, in my view, a pretty nor a hopeful one. Having first adopted and moved towards network governance, the PHN – presumably at the urging of, and certainly with the support of the Council of Deputy Ministers of Health to which it reports – has moved more towards 'institutional simplification', a strategy which is described herein as "untenable" and "inadequate", and as noted above, has backed away from a more inclusive partnership with the non-government world. I can testify to the accuracy of Claude's history (which is to say, I suppose, that I share his perceptions and biases). I share his concerns with the effects of the reorganization of the Public Health Network, specifically the reduced flexibility, more structure and control and – of particular concern to me – the exclusion of non-governmental voices at the table, or put another way, the restriction of discussions and decisions to government departments and staff alone.

Reading this book, one can see why the government might want to back away from network governance. Its implications are quite radical, even revolutionary, and clearly threatening to a centralist and controlling worldview. Claude writes in chapter 8, for example, that "No longer is it acceptable to govern as if all power is vested in the public authority;" that we need new forms of accountability because "[T]he type of accountability that reflects a linear, mono-centric type of structure is no longer appropriate," that the current rule-driven federal public service "has made it almost impossible to play by the rules and achieve significant results," and that we need public servants who play a more active role, who are "virtuous schemers" and are working (citing Box et al. 2001) to improve "the quality of democracy by actively helping people govern themselves." Heady stuff indeed!

But if Claude and the many authors from whose works he draws are correct, this step backwards may be only a hiccup on the road to network governance, because perhaps, when the centre cannot hold, it is what will stand between us and mere anarchy being loosed upon the world.

Dr. Trevor Hancock
Professor and Senior Scholar
School of Public Health and Social policy
University of Victoria

January 2012

"Let all men know how empty and worthless is the power of kings."

– King Canute, 11th century

INTRODUCTION

GOVERNANCE, NETWORKS AND PUBLIC HEALTH

Why a book about public health governance in Canada? There are two main reasons. To begin with, public health, and sometimes the lack of it, continues to challenge our society. There is nothing new about infectious diseases. Plagues have been chronicled for thousands of years. The Bubonic Plague of the mid-14th century is perhaps the strongest in our consciousness of an "ancient" infectious disease pandemic. The influenza pandemic of 1918-19, which killed an estimated 50 to 100 million people worldwide, is still alive in our collective memories. More recently, the world was jolted out of its infectious disease complacency by two events: the SARS crisis of 2003 and the H1N1 pandemic of 2009. Although the two recent events did not take many lives, relatively speaking, they served as powerful reminders that even with our advanced technology and knowledge, infectious diseases have not been "conquered." On the contrary, new strains are constantly emerging and, assisted by the global movement of people, can be transmitted around the world in a matter of hours.

It is not just infectious diseases that pose threats to our health. Globally, non-communicable diseases, or chronic diseases, such as cancer, cardiovascular disease, respiratory diseases, diabetes, neurological diseases, to name a few, are the cause of far more premature deaths than infectious diseases (World Health Organization 2003b, chapter 1: 8) Moreover, the incidence of such diseases is, in many cases, increasing, particularly in low and middle income countries. Reduction in the use of tobacco in developed countries has been one of the few clear advances of the past decades but, even here, it is a battle the must continue to be fought to counter the subtle and not so subtle manipulations of the tobacco industry. The most recent threat to emerge is the obesity pandemic which has struck North America particularly hard, and is gaining ground in most parts of the world. Behavioural, social, environmental and physiological causes are all identified as key "risk factors" but we still have no effective strategy to control the incidence of obesity. Until a way is found to curb this trend, the rates of many of the chronic diseases mentioned above will continue to rise, at substantial cost to the economies of states and, more important, to people's lives.

This is not to paint an overly gloomy a picture; life expectancy continues to increase in high income countries, though much needs to be done elsewhere. Rather, it is to say that public health as a discipline is at least as relevant as ever, arguably even more so, and the difficulties it faces are growing. Effective responses are needed for the problems we are facing, and how we organize ourselves for doing so is crucial. This brings us to the second reason to examine public health governance: this aspect of public health, in Canada and elsewhere, is too often over-shadowed in favour of the more technical or scientific aspects. Much of the public health literature has focused on documenting the nature and causes of health threats and proposing ways to deal with these threats, whether through the development or use of a vaccine, or anti-viral or, more broadly, through a campaign to educate the public on the importance of hand-washing, physical activity, healthy eating and so on. However, insufficient attention has been paid to how those objectives are to be realized from a policy process perspective. As will be discussed below, public health is a very broad field that touches on many different areas and involves a diverse cross-section of actors and organizations. The simple, yet deeply perplexing question is how to bring about and maintain the collaboration of these myriad actors towards a common set of objectives. In a 1985 article, Harlan Cleveland put the core question of modern governance plainly when he asked: "How do you get everybody in on the act and still get some action?" (Cleveland 1985: 189). As it relates to public health, there is more urgency to the question now than ever.

A frequent subject of discussion in public health circles is how to translate 'evidence' to policy. There is often an assumption in these discussions that the appropriate policy outcomes will occur naturally if public health experts can provide clear and irrefutable evidence of the seriousness of a particular health threat, or the advisability of a certain course of action. However, as many students of the public policy process have demonstrated, the relationship between evidence and policy is anything but linear, and the process involved is indeed multi-faceted and often far 'messier' than might be the case in a perfectly Cartesian world (see, for example, Kingdon 2003; Sabatier 1988; Mintrom and Vergari 1996). Central questions to be asked include: How does one achieve those health outcomes that necessarily depend on the active participation of others? Who leads in such exercises? What does it mean to lead? What incentives are there for others to 'follow'?

The purpose of this book is to examine public health governance in Canada, with a particular focus on the use, misuse and opportunities presented by networks in public health. In this way, the book would be of interest to public health practitioners who wish to find ways to maximize the impact of their activities, as well as to students of governance who seek more specific applications of the concept of network governance. The importance of networks and partnerships in public health is often acknowledged, not least by the Chief Public Health Officer, who stated in his 2008 report that "it takes the combined effort of networks both within and outside the public health system to address population-wide health challenges" (Public Health Agency of Canada 2008: 8). Unfortunately, this core aspect of the governance of public health in Canada has too seldom been critically examined or analyzed. Networks, for all their complexities and ambiguities, are central to public health governance in Canada, and a more systematic understanding and rigorous application of these mechanisms is needed to confront the public health challenges of the future.

The central proposition of this book can be stated as follows. First, as in many other sectors, public health has witnessed a transition from government to governance, implying broader, more inclusive decision-making structures related to public policy. This shift has been driven by the level of complexity presented by the vast range of issues with which public health must grapple. Second, it will be argued that network governance, tailored to suit the particular circumstances in place, is needed to address these modern-day challenges. Unfortunately, the mechanisms that have been put in place at the national level are not adequate to meet the challenges that present themselves. Finally, we argue that the changes required are at both the cultural and structural levels. In other words, it is not simply a question of putting the 'right' mechanisms in place. These must be accompanied by a shared understanding of, and commitment to, being in the 'business' of addressing the challenges posed by public health through networks, and an appreciation and application of the skills and personal competencies that are needed to make this work. In a nutshell, this book is a plea for a more deliberate and rigorous application of a network governance regime in all facets of public health in Canada.

The book is divided in four parts. The first part will seek to set the stage for the discussion that follows. In the first chapter, we will define, in more precise terms, what might be called the governance challenges in public health. In this chapter, we will discuss the fragmented state of public health in Canada, and how this inhibits collaboration and coordination. Policy and organizational fragmentation, of course, is not unique to public health. The point remains, however, that finding a way to accomplish public health objectives in a fragmented environment is the core of the issue to be addressed.

The first chapter will examine this question in terms of three 'fault lines,' specifically, *the intergovernmental divides, the intersectoral challenges, and the government-civil society relationships.* From an intergovernmental perspective, public health federalism is necessarily a key aspect, since Canada's federal regime affects, and often shapes, many public policy issues in Canada, and public health is no exception. At the same time, since much of the 'action' in public health takes place at the community level, the relationship between provincial governments, which have primary legislative authority in the area, and the local level, is also pivotal. Next, public health, to be effective, must go outside the health area, narrowly defined, and reach many other policy sectors and, therefore, the relationships between public health and other departments and agencies within the same government are crucial. In many cases, the interdepartmental gap within governments can be as difficult to bridge as the intergovernmental divides. Finally, as has been noted, public health is not just about the actions of governments. On the contrary, civil society, in the form of non-governmental organizations and private sector organizations, has a huge impact on public health policy and programs in Canada. Taken together, the discussion of these three fault lines will try to shed light on the difficulties posed by fragmentation in the public health sector in Canada, as a first step to finding a model to overcome these challenges.

The second chapter will look at the potential offered by network governance to address the fault lines described in the previous chapter. If fragmentation is 'the problem,' is network governance 'the solution'? There is no simple answer to this question, but before we can begin to answer it, we must establish what we mean by the term. Of course, network governance has been understood in many ways, and it is beyond the scope of this book to attempt to conduct a comprehensive review. Our main objective in this chapter will be to discuss in broad terms what is meant by network governance and review briefly its key characteristics, in order to establish the basis for the discussion to follow.

Part II will attempt to situate the discussion in specific contexts. Public health is a broad concept, and as such operates in a wide array of spheres, or 'theatres,' each with its specific set of governance requirements. For this reason, the following three chapters will examine three such theatres: the Pan-Canadian Public Health Network (PHN); the emergency preparedness and response context; and the Canadian Heart Health Initiative (CHHI). The purpose of these reviews is to examine the governance dimension in each one of these cases and to discuss how a network governance model, more systematically applied, could lead to more inclusive, effective and sustainable policy outcomes.

Chapter 3 will discuss the PHN as the key piece of network infrastructure at the national level. The architecture of the PHN contains both conventional and non-conventional features. On the one hand, it functions very much like a conventional federal/provincial/territorial committee (FPT) which can be found in many other policy sectors. In other respects, however, it departs from the conventional, for example, by including members outside government, mostly university researchers. While the PHN might be seen as an attempt to move in the direction of network governance, this chapter will argue that the network infrastructure established in 2005 falls short of what is needed for a truly inclusive, collaborative approach. Moreover, we will argue that the set of major reforms to the PHN, which were approved in 2010 following a review of its operation and are being implemented at the time of writing, may actually represent a step away from what is needed to make network governance a functioning reality.

Chapter 4 will review the functioning of networks in public health emergency situations, using the SARS crisis of 2003 and the H1N1 pandemic of 2009 as the context. As appealing as the concept of network governance may sound in theory, what is to be done in an emergency situation, such as in the event of a pandemic, when quick decisions and efficient execution are paramount? Is network governance feasible in 'war-time,' or must it be put on hold, at least temporarily, in favour of a command and control structure to deal with the crisis? Much of the literature assessing the SARS events in Canada, in particular four major reports – two at the national level, and two commissioned by the Ontario government – and much of the secondary literature on the subject, recommend reverting to more top-down approaches to deal with such crises in the future. Put simply, the argument appears to be that while networks are appropriate for 'peace-time' situations, in times of public health emergencies what is required is a command-and-control structure led by a commander-in-chief – some refer to a public health 'czar'– with the power and authority to override the fragmented policy and organizational environment. We will challenge this view, and argue that the network governance model need not be abandoned to deal with public health crises, although more centralized forms of network governance may be needed in these circumstances. Indeed, while 'institutional simplification' may seem attractive at first blush, it may ultimately lead to exactly the opposite type of outcome from what is intended or required.

Chapter 5 presents a case study of the Canadian Heart Health Initiative (CHHI) as an example of a 'peace-time' initiative. The CHHI is an initiative which operated for almost 20 years with the objective of improving heart health in Canada, and which involved Health Canada, at the federal level, provincial governments, and a large number of voluntary sector organizations (VSOs). Although it was not conceptualized as such in its day, the CHHI provides a sort of 'natural experiment' of network governance. Because of its intergovernmental (both federal/provincial and provincial/local), inter-sectoral, and extra-governmental dimensions, it effectively sought to bridge the three fault lines identified earlier. In this way, the CHHI provides an excellent learning opportunity, both from the perspectives of where it was successful, and where it fell short.

Part III is all about expanding the base of relationships that are necessary for a broader model of governance. In chapter 6, we will examine the role of civil society and, in particular, the voluntary sector, to shed light on how players from this sector participate in the policy process. The term 'partnerships' is commonly used in this sector, but it is important to ask how the relationships between governments and voluntary sector organizations can be understood more precisely and to what extent they are consistent with a network governance approach. Following a review of a number of specific cases in the public health sector, including some which span across more than one category, our conclusion is that while there have been some recent departures from the norm, it is highly questionable whether the relationships in place are conducive to network governance.

It is also important to situate public health governance in the global context. As has often been said, public health threats, whether in the form of infectious or non-infectious diseases, do not respect national borders. This is not new, and the forces of globalization have greatly accelerated the movement around the world of people and goods, with all that comes with it. In chapter 7, we will argue that the pressures for more collaborative and inclusive forms of governance are mirrored at the global level. What previously was the preserve of states, working through international institutions such as the World Health Organization (WHO) and its regional bodies, has now been broadened to include non-state organizations much more directly than previously. To illustrate this point, we will review the experience and impact of three recent (post 2000) global developments related to public health. These are: the WHO handling of the SARS crisis of 2003; the process leading up to the Framework Agreement on Tobacco Control; and the Global Strategy on Diet, Physical Activity and Health. All three reflect an important change in global models of governance in public health, which some authors have described as a shift from international health governance to global health governance (see Dodgson et al. 2002). This trend has important implications for public health in Canada. Key issues, such as accountability, legitimacy, evaluation, transparency and monitoring, with appropriate modifications, apply to both global and domestic contexts. Furthermore, the skills necessary to

make these mechanisms work in practice are applicable to both
environments. Canada, as a player in these processes, can both
contribute to, and learn from, the new collaborative governance
mechanisms that are developing on the world stage. Perhaps
most fundamentally, the global shift to more collaborative forms
of governance empowers a broader range of players who, in turn,
will expect to play a meaningful role in the policy process at the
domestic level.

The focus of Part IV will be on the practicalities of making
network governance viable. To some, network governance may
sound somewhat naive and utopian. Is the search for the answer
to Cleveland's question, cited earlier, ultimately an exercise in
futility? How realistic is it to expect that broad social consensus
can be achieved around complex issues in the presence of so
many competing and entrenched interests? Chapter 8 attempts
to take stock of three main issues that must be addressed before
network governance can achieve its full potential in the public
health sector in Canada. The first deals with the issue of the
'workability' of network governance, and discusses how this
can be achieved through the use of 'metagovernance.' The second
question relates to the challenge of how the interconnected
concepts of accountability, legitimacy and transparency can be
incorporated into workable forms of network governance. Finally,
we examine whether and how network governance in public
health can flourish within the formal hierarchical structure of a
Westminster-style parliamentary democracy.

The final chapter deals with what it would mean to establish
a network governance regime in public health. This chapter will
propose three building blocks to help achieve this objective. To
use a sports metaphor, one must know the nature of the game
one is playing, understand its basic rules, and possess the key
competencies to play the game successfully. Essentially this
speaks to the need to develop and nurture a *culture* in public
health which is conducive to collaborative forms of governance,
combined with the strategies and skills which are necessary to
achieve success. This chapter will explore the practical steps that
can be taken to establish the foundation for a network governance
regime in public health.

The study of networks does not lend itself to formulaic
language. Given the extreme variety of contexts and circumstances
in which modern governance is situated, it will be difficult to

achieve a high level of predictability of results. Much remains to be learned about specifically what works best in what circumstances. Still, useful insights can be gleaned from the literature that can help practitioners increase their chances of success. Furthermore, although the focus of this study is on public health, the conclusions one draws can be applied to other sectors as well, with appropriate contextual modifications. By studying particular applications, we will hopefully be able to find insights and suggestions that can be applied more broadly.

The source material used for this study is a combination of document review and interviews with key individuals. As much as possible, I drew from publicly available literature in the form of primary sources, such as government reports, as well as secondary literature. In many cases, it proved extremely helpful to supplement the documentary evidence with interviews with key informants. In all, 56 interviews were carried out. These interviews were semi-structured, in that they were initiated on the basis of specific questions, but were flexible enough to follow the interviewee in areas that were not originally anticipated but that proved to be very valuable. To encourage candour, they were held on a strictly confidential, not-for-attribution basis. In order to respect the confidentiality of the interviews, they will be referenced in the book by number, accompanied by the date on which the interview took place.

Finally, on a personal note, I benefitted from my experience as Director General of the Centre for Health Promotion at the Public Health Agency of Canada (PHAC) from 2001 to 2008. It was particularly fascinating to be part of the management team of the Population and Public Health Branch of Health Canada during the SARS crisis, and the *'prise de conscience'* around public health which followed, culminating in that branch being transformed into the Public Health Agency of Canada. Between 2008 and 2010, I was fortunate enough to be able to research this book as Visiting Fellow at the Graduate School of Public and International Affairs at the University of Ottawa, which provided a unique opportunity to combine those years as a practitioner with research findings. There is much left to be learned, and it is hoped that this book will contribute in some small way to a discussion that will lead to new understandings and insights.

In many ways, a book is a team project, and this one is no exception. To begin with, I wish to thank David Butler-Jones,

Jane Billings and Sylvie Stachenko at the Public Health Agency of Canada, for agreeing to and supporting my Interchange arrangement with the University of Ottawa during which time this book was conceived and written. I am also grateful to the staff at the Canada School for Public Service for facilitating this arrangement. François Houle, former Dean of Social Sciences and subsequently, Vice-President Academic at the University of Ottawa, and Luc Juillet, former Director of the Graduate School of Public and International Affairs, supported my arrival at the university and made me feel welcome during my stay. David Zussman, holder of the Jarislowsky Chair in Public Sector Management and current Director of the GSPIA, was a consistent source of encouragement, insight and sound advice. Many thanks are due to the dozens of individuals who generously gave of their time to be interviewed for this book. Without exception, these individuals were candid, forthcoming and patient in answering the questions I put to them. I have tried my best to accurately represent their views and perspectives. Ron St. John, Dick de Jong, Theresa Tam, Claude Giroux, Patrick Fafard, David McLean, Bill Jeffrey, Joe McDonald and Elinor Wilson reviewed chapters at various stages of production and provided valuable comments. Michel Sleiman, my research assistant at the University of Ottawa, carried out helpful bibliographic searches and literature reviews and assisted with many of the interviews.

I am especially grateful to Gilles Paquet, Professor Emeritus at the University of Ottawa, senior editor of Invenire Books, and passionate advocate for collaborative governance. Without his support, coaching and inspiration, this book would not have been possible.

I would also like to thank Ruth Hubbard of Invenire Books for her helpful comments on the manuscript, and McEvoy Galbreath and her team for their careful work in copyediting this book.

Finally, I wish to thank Anna DeHart, my wife and partner, for being unfailingly encouraging, supportive and understanding during the period it took me to research and write this book.

Notwithstanding the very considerable help and support I received, all omissions, inaccuracies, and misinterpretations are mine alone.

I – SETTING THE STAGE

CHAPTER 1

PUBLIC HEALTH AND FRAGMENTATION:
THREE FAULT LINES

Introduction

Benjamin Disraeli once stated: "The health of the people is really the foundation upon which all their happiness and all their power as a state depends." In stating this, Disraeli was implicitly acknowledging the importance of the public health system as an area of public policy. At the risk of stating the obvious, without good health, a society cannot prosper. Yet as important as "the health of the people" is, the public health system in Canada performs at a sub-optimal level, diminished by its internal divisions. This system is frequently characterized as being fragmented and in need of greater coordination and integration (Butler-Jones 2009: I-1). Indeed, the theme of fragmentation runs through much of the literature about public health, not only in Canada, but also globally. But what precisely is meant by fragmentation and why should this be considered a serious problem? Some level of fragmentation could probably be associated with most policy sectors in a modern society, and more particularly in a state, like Canada, with a federal system of government. What is at the root of this concern about fragmentation and, more specifically, what does it mean for governance in the public health sector?

In this chapter, we will attempt to describe in more precise terms how fragmentation in public health manifests itself in Canada, the reasons for it, and why this is seen as particularly problematic from a governance perspective. Public health, by its very nature, inevitably cuts across a number of jurisdictions, policy areas and social sectors. In this context, we will discuss three major 'fault lines' in public health that have presented obstacles to achieving a greater level of coordination and collaboration. The first refers to the 'intergovernmental' divides. The sharpest of these, not surprisingly, is the jurisdictional separation between the federal and the provincial (and territorial) orders of government. This also includes the distinction between provincial and local levels, which in public health is of very real importance. Beyond this, there is also the 'inter-sectoral' divide, that is, the division that occurs within jurisdictions – federal, provincial-territorial, and even local – between different policy and program areas that have an impact on the health of populations. Finally, 'government-civil society' relations are also germane because of the increasingly important role of voluntary sector organizations (VSOs), in particular, not only in delivering programs and services on behalf of government, but also as important players in setting public policy.

Seen together, the end result of these fault lines is that coordination necessarily becomes a challenge to overcome, to put it mildly, with direct (negative) consequences for the health of Canadians. However, as Disraeli said in another instance: "Despair is the conclusion of fools." Coming to grips with the nature of the problem allows for an exploration of possible remedial actions that might be taken. We will argue in the following chapter that collaborative governance and, specifically network governance, appropriately applied and nurtured, may provide such a course of action.

The length and breadth of public health

Before going further, we need to define the terms we are using, since both 'public health' and 'governance' are subject to a range of interpretations and misinterpretations. Unfortunately, 'public health' is often confused with publicly funded health care, despite the fact that these are two very different concepts. A classic definition of public health was provided by J.M. Last, who wrote that public health is "the set of efforts organized by society to protect, promote and restore people's health through collective and social action" (Last 1998: 6). Whereas health 'care' operates primarily at the clinical level, involving a relationship between the health care provider and the individual, the focus of public health is at the societal level. While there is an area where public health and the provision of health care intersect, the field on which public health must play extends far beyond the health sector.

The main conclusion one draws from Last's definition is the broad area covered by public health. There are, of course, some aspects that pertain to public health in the narrow sense, such as immunization but, beyond these, there is a whole range of issues that fall outside what would normally be seen as the health field. *A New Perspective on the Health of Canadians,* known as the *Lalonde Report* of 1974, was a seminal document in Canada, pointing out that public health did not depend only on physicians and nurses and hospitals, as many assumed, but had much deeper social roots (Lalonde 1974: 18). This thinking was subsequently reflected in the *Ottawa Charter on Health Promotion* of 1986, which stated that "health promotion is not just the responsibility of the health sector, but goes beyond healthy life-styles to well-being." The *Ottawa Charter's* depiction of health, as "a positive concept emphasizing social and personal resources, as well as physical capacities," served to underline how public health had to be seen as the business of all of society. Most recently, the *Bangkok Charter for Health Promotion in a Globalized World* of 2005 reflected the same concept of health and added to the critical factors affecting health such issues as: increasing inequalities within and between countries; new patterns of consumption and communication; commercialization; global environmental change; and urbanization.

Looked at in this way, health pertains in some way to most endeavours of society. Dr. Elinor Wilson, former head of the Canadian Public Health Association, once commented publicly that "public health is everything!" Admittedly, the connection with some policy areas is more direct in some cases than in others. In Canada, early public health efforts dealt with agricultural practices related to food safety, such as the pasteurization of milk, as well as environmental issues related to water quality and waste disposal. Quarantine and immunization issues, and the containment of cholera and smallpox epidemics, also featured prominently. By the beginning of the 20th century, more attention was paid to maternal and child health, child development and nutrition (Mowat and de Jong 2003: 22). Together, these form what one might call the inner circle of public health issues. Since about the middle of the 20th century, however, as the focus of public health shifted from infectious diseases to chronic diseases, there has been a broadening of the scope of public health in the direction of "healthy public policy," referring to the less obvious issues that nonetheless have a direct impact on public health (Turnock and Atchison 2002). For example, these now include urban infrastructure and transportation policy, given the influence these areas can have in providing incentives or disincentives to being physically active. Similarly, tax policy and trade subsidies can have an impact on whether people choose healthy foods or others. Industrial policy can also determine whether hazardous products are allowed to enter the marketplace, potentially increasing risks of illness or injury.

The last portion of the 20th century and the beginning of the 21st saw an increasing interest in the social determinants of health. The link between poverty and health, and between social inequalities and health, is not new, and in fact has been widely acknowledged at least since the 19th century. In its report, *Closing the Gap in a Generation* (World Health Organization 2008a), the WHO's Commission on the Social Determinants of Health, led by Sir Michael Marmot, signalled a heightening interest in documenting the relationships and proposing strategies to counter the negative impact of poverty and social inequalities on health.

Public health practitioners, then, work on a broad canvas which leads to a complex web of relationships. In some cases, where the issue is more clearly seen as health-related, they find themselves playing a leading role. In many other cases, where the issue pertains more directly to another policy area, but with important implications for health, they must attempt to influence the outcome of the discussion, recognizing that the ultimate decision will be taken outside the public health arena. In both cases, however, they must work with and through others to achieve their ultimate objectives of "promoting health, preventing disease, and prolonging life."

Three major fault lines

It is to be expected, given the above, that divisions – which we will call fault lines – should occur within this panoply of relationships. In the final analysis, the crucial question is how can these divisions be bridged in the interests of protecting and improving the health of the population? Before attempting to answer this question, we must first examine the nature of these cleavages. The following section will identify where the major divisions occur.

The intergovernmental divides

By far the sharpest fault line in public health in Canada, and one that has received the most attention in the literature, relates to the relationships between the federal government and provincial/ territorial governments, or what some observers have called "public health federalism" (Wilson and Lazar 2008). In the final report of the Royal Commission on the Future of Health Care in Canada, Commissioner Roy Romanow remarked on "the mutual respect and trust that has been missing in recent years, particularly in the relationship between the federal and provincial governments, and among the various actors in the health care system" (Romanow 2002: 46). He went on to say that the intergovernmental mechanisms for addressing health issues had become "increasingly dysfunctional and characterized by fractious debate" among the federal, provincial and territorial governments (FPT) governments. Romanow was referring primarily to issues relating to the health 'care' system in making these comments, and one would need to temper them somewhat in applying them to the public health system. The type of federal-provincial squabbling over funding that one saw in the 1990s and early in 2000s did not reflect themselves to the same extent over public health issues. This is perhaps because the financial stakes were not nearly as high in the latter case, considering that it is estimated that public health represents only approximately two percent of the overall expenditures on health in Canada (Lozon and Alikhan 2007: 55).

Still, Romanow's comments have resonance in the context of public health. Although the level of bickering might be lower historically, there has been considerable evidence of a lack of coordination. The *Naylor Report*, which looked at the SARS events with a view of assessing what had gone wrong in the response of governments to this infectious disease, and what could be done to improve the capacity of governments to respond to threats to public health in the future, stated that: "Our first theme is that the single largest impediment to dealing successfully with future public health crises is the lack of a collaborative framework and ethos among different levels of government" (National Advisory

Committee on SARS and Public Health 2003: 212). In its review of the public health system in Canada, the Institute of Population and Public Health of the Canadian Institutes of Health Research (CIHR) concluded critically that it was, in fact, inaccurate to refer to a public health 'system' in Canada. Instead, the report stated, it would be more accurate to describe the situation in Canada as "a grouping of multiple systems with varying roles, strengths and linkages" (Canadian Institutes for Health Research 2003: 17). Similarly, Jennifer Keelan, who looked at immunization policy in Canada, referred to "systemic problems with Canadian public health governance whereby each jurisdiction works largely in isolation to determine critical public health policies, such as disease surveillance, program planning, and evaluation" (Keelan 2008: 8).

To a certain extent, these disconnects are rooted in the constitutional ambiguities around the responsibility for public health in Canada. This has been closely examined in other works (Braën 2002; Jackman 2000), so there is no need to treat this issue in detail here. At the most general level, the key point is that "there is no clear authority over public health in the Canadian constitution" (Wilson and Lazar 2008; Jackman 2000). Stated otherwise, both federal and provincial governments have the legislative authority to act in various aspects of public health (Braën 2002: vi).

Provincial governments, which are recognized as being the primary players in public health, derive their authority in the area from the provisions in the *Constitution Act, 1867* relating to: the establishment, maintenance, and management of hospitals (s. 92.7); matters of a local or private nature (s. 92.16); property and civil rights (s. 92.13); and education (s. 93) (Braën 2002: 7). For its part, the federal government draws its authority in the area from its ability to legislate in the area of criminal law; from the use of its spending power; and from its authority to ensure peace, order and good government (Braën 2002: 10). It also has specific authority to make laws respecting quarantine matters (s. 91.11). Parliament's authority in the matter of criminal law gives it the legislative authority to act in matters respecting the manufacture, sale and distribution of products posing a risk to public health. This can include food labelling, restrictions on tobacco, and regulation of products posing a risk to children (Braën 2002: 11). The peace, order and good government provision, for its part, provides the basis for the federal government's use of emergency powers (Braën 2002: 13). In addition, the federal government also has the legislative authority to act in matters relating to the health of veterans, members of the armed forces, and the health needs of First Nations and Inuit people (Braën 2002: 14).

In practice, however, the field of public health is characterized by a considerable amount of ambiguity about roles and responsibilities which has set the scene for federal/provincial/ territorial tensions, if not outright conflicts. This can be driven by differences of priority between jurisdictions due to varying regional needs and circumstances and perhaps ideologies. While certain issues may be high on the list of concerns of one jurisdiction, this might not be shared by others. This can be particularly problematic when the contributions of both orders of government are necessary for the success of a particular initiative. This is typically the case around issues such as immunization, chronic disease prevention, health promotion and emergency preparedness, where the provincial infrastructure is necessary to reach the target audience, but where federal government intervention is often expected for purposes of standard setting, research, evaluation methodologies and, particularly, funding. Kumanan Wilson (2004: 410) identifies three emerging challenges in the public health policy arena that have the potential to undermine program delivery due to conflict between the orders of government. These relate to:

- Externalities and spill-overs: refers to finding ways to deal with threats to health in one region that could spill over to other regions;
- Funding disputes: occur when one order of government (usually provincial/territorial) has responsibility in an area, but lacks a revenue source; and
- Data-sharing: has been a consistent source of tension between the federal government and many provincial and territorial governments, and one over which the Auditor General of Canada has expressed concern in three separate reports (1999, 2002 and 2008).

This is not to suggest that collaboration cannot or does not occur between orders of government in public health. Students of Canadian federalism have written about 'collaborative federalism,' meaning "the process by which national goals are achieved, not by the federal government acting alone, or by the federal government shaping provincial behaviour through the exercise of its spending power, but by some or all of the 11 governments and the territories acting collectively" (Cameron and Simeon 2002: 54). To be sure, there are a number of examples of collaborative federalism manifesting itself in public health. The Health Goals for Canada, for example, were agreed to in October, 2005, through a consensus-driven process involving federal/provincial/territorial governments without any financial inducement by the federal government. These goals are meant to "provide a tool to guide further action on the determinants of health and help to strengthen the management of horizontal issues" (Public Health Agency of Canada, *Health Goals for Canada* website). Similarly, the Pan-Canadian Healthy Living Strategy of 2005 was negotiated through an intensive and mostly collegial federal/provincial/territorial process that did not involve federal inducements or financial commitments. Both were formally approved by the federal government and all provinces and territories (with the exception of Quebec) at the ministerial level. Admittedly, these initiatives are examples of policy alignment rather than programmatic initiatives, and do not have either direct cost implications or enforcement mechanisms. However, the Healthy Living Strategy contains specific targets for improvements in healthy eating, physical activity, and healthy weights by 2015, and the federal/provincial/territorial governments will need to report publically on their success or failure to reach those targets, including providing joint annual progress reports on their work in relation to these targets (*Integrated Pan-Canadian Healthy Living Strategy* 2005).

The development of the National Immunization Strategy is another case in point. Immunization policy was identified in the 2002 Report of the Commission on the Future of Health Care in Canada, commonly known as the *Romanow Report,* as requiring a higher level of collaboration between federal, provincial and territorial governments than was evident at that time. The report stated that the lack of joint planning between governments made Canada ill-prepared "to face new and emerging problems due to globalization and the evolution of infectious diseases" (Romanow 2002: 134). Indeed, immunization policy at that time followed a checker-board pattern, with different provincial and territorial practices on which vaccines to cover through public health insurance, the number of doses to administer, and the age at which they were given, often at variation with the recommendations of the federally appointed National Advisory Committee on Immunization (Keelan 2008: 9).

To address this issue, federal, provincial and territorial governments agreed to a National Immunization Strategy (NIS) in 2003. A key feature of this was a federal government allocation of $400 million in the form of an *ad hoc* third party trust, from which the provinces and territories could draw, most of which was targeted for the implementation of four vaccines which had recently been recommended (Keelan 2008: 14). Furthermore, in 2004, the Canadian Immunization Committee was established to implement the NIS. This committee includes representatives from the federal government and all provincial and territorial jurisdictions, and makes recommendations based on a joint decision-making process (Keelan 2008: 18). These recommendations are then presented to federal/provincial/ territorial committees, which are part of the Public Health Network (see chapter 3) dealing with infectious diseases, and eventually to the Conference of the Deputy Ministers of Health. This approach to the NIS is generally seen as a success, and has been suggested as a model to follow in other areas of public health (Keelan 2008: 27; Keelan et al. 2008).

Certain factors probably increase the likelihood of federal/ provincial/territorial collaboration in public health issues. For example, collaboration may be more likely at the middle or lower levels of organizations and around operational or programmatic issues. Peters has observed that "co-ordination is often a function of negotiations among the lower echelons of organizations around specific issues or clients" (Peters 1998: 307). Referring to the Canadian context, Armstrong and Lenihan observe that collaborative culture becomes "more and more difficult to realize the further up the hierarchy one travelled" (Armstrong and Lenihan 1999: 30).

Moreover, collaboration is more likely at the program level than at the strategic level of government agencies and departments. Cameron and Simeon point out that the high levels of mutual distrust in federal/provincial/territorial relations is "much more evident at the level of first ministers and their central agencies than it is among line ministers and officials, who are more likely to share policy goals and political constituencies" (Cameron and Simeon 2002: 68). Angus and

Bégin (2000) substantiate this point as it applies to federal/
provincial/territorial health ministers conferences:

>...*above all, what is definitely hindering their [FPT health
minsters conferences] success is the active participation of
intergovernmental affairs officials 'guiding' or instructing
provincial ministers (or the federal one) as to what is acceptable
and what is not, for it turns the process into a competitive
constitutional match at the expense of the problem under
consideration* (Angus and Bégin 2000: 182).[1]

In a similar vein, Johns et al. distinguish between intergovernmental relations (IGR) which takes place at the more
strategic level and involves officials in intergovernmental
affairs, ministers and central agencies, and intergovernmental
management (IGM), which involves departmental officials and
functions more at the programmatic level (Johns et al. 2006:
631). Essentially, their point is that strong intergovernmental
relationships, and indeed consensus, are more likely in the IGM
context than in IGR. Those at the departmental level will be far
more likely to frame the issues in which they are involved in a
similar way, and to share a perspective on what the objectives
should be from a public policy perspective. Other students of
federal/provincial/territorial relations in Canada have arrived
at a similar conclusion (see Dupré 1987 and Lazar 2006).

Finally, the impact of "epistemic communities" is also an
important factor contributing to collaboration in the area of public
health. These have been defined as "a network of professionals
with recognized expertise and competence in a particular domain
and an authoritative claim to policy-relevant knowledge
within that domain or issue area" (Haas 1992: 3). Public health
organizations typically employ a high number of employees:
physicians, nurses or individuals who have backgrounds in a
health-related field, such as epidemiology, nutrition, human
kinesiology, veterinary science and so on. These individuals
will often continue to belong to professional associations in their
fields of expertise, such as the Canadian Medical Association,
the Canadian Nurses Association, and the Dieticians of Canada.
Many will also share memberships in organizations such as
the Canadian Public Health Association and other networks of

[1] Monique Bégin, as a former federal Minister of Health, would have a particular
perspective on this dynamic.

public health practitioners. Although specific documentation about epistemic communities in public health is lacking, it can be expected that the common values and perspectives derived from a common professional formation, as well as membership in these organizations, would go some distance in counter-balancing the federal/provincial/territorial cleavages discussed above. A case in point is the Council of Chief Medical Officers of Health (CCMOH), which will be discussed in greater detail in chapter 3. The CCMOH, a federal/provincial/territorial committee, which is responsible for providing technical advice to the Public Health Network, is entirely composed of physicians, representing the Public Health Agency of Canada and each of the 13 provincial and territorial jurisdictions. When dealing with substantive public health issues, the priorities and concerns of the jurisdiction they represent will be balanced (although not necessarily neutralized) with the common professional training and outlook they share (Interview #1: May 9, 2011).

Notwithstanding the existence of a level of federal/provincial/territorial collaboration in public health matters, the overall conclusion remains that public health federalism remains a major fault line affecting efforts to address public health issues in Canada. Although one can point to examples of collaborative federalism, these tend to be episodic and *ad hoc*, rather than systematic. As can be said for collaborative federalism in general, these relationships are likely to ebb and flow with the times (Cameron and Simeon 2002: 65). Often, as in the case of the Healthy Living Strategy, they are dependent on the good relations and trust between the participants (Interview #2: September 29, 2010). A change in the level of commitment by the governments in office, or even among the key individuals involved, can lead to the initiative being side-tracked or shelved. Since there is no legislative base or formal decision-making rules, such undertakings are bound to be somewhat fragile (Cameron and Simeon 2002: 64). As Deber et al. put it:

> *Co-operation in public health is largely based on voluntary agreements, and the federal government remains reluctant to compel co-operation. With respect to health promotion, this is often wasteful and has long-term consequences in terms of foregone benefits. With regard to potential pandemics, however, it could be disastrous; infectious agents are unlikely to respect provincial/territorial boundaries* (Deber et al. 2007: 69-70).

As will be discussed in chapter 4, there are consequences for attempting "to compel co-operation." At this point, we merely wish to draw attention to the divisive impact, potential and real, of federal/provincial/territorial relations on the public health enterprise in Canada.

The intergovernmental fault line does not only impact federal/provincial/territorial relations. The provincial/local government relationships can prove to be equally challenging. It is often recognized that what happens at the local level is the "backbone" of the public health system (Wilson and Lazar 2005: 17). Yet broad policy directions come largely from the relevant provincial/territorial government agencies. This can lead to fairly complex relationships that require considerable coordination. As will be discussed in greater detail in chapter 4, the reports on the SARS events commissioned by the Government of Ontario provide important insight into these relationships during the pre-SARS period. Both the *Campbell Report* and the *Walker Report* document in detail the break-down in communication between the provincial and the local levels during the SARS crisis, and the damaging impact this had on attempting to respond to the crisis. Indeed, many of the core recommendations found in both reports revolve around how to re-structure governance in public health in Ontario and, particularly, as it relates to the respective roles of the province vis-à-vis the local and regional bodies.

While many of the recommendations in the *Campbell Report* and the *Walker Report* are in the direction of strengthening the province's hand in dealing with local authorities, authorities at the local level tend to guard their own autonomy, and underscore the importance of basing their interventions and partnerships on the circumstances that exist "on the ground" (Interview #3: December 23, 2010; Lozon and Alikhan 2007: 57-58). Effective relationships at the local level are crucial during infectious disease outbreaks, so that effective communication can take place with clinics, hospitals and private practitioners. Although of a less urgent nature, strong community relationships will also be necessary in attempting to prevent non-communicable diseases, where partnerships need to be struck with schools, municipal governments and a range of voluntary sector organizations to reduce the incidence of injuries and to encourage tobacco cessation, breast-feeding, physical activity, healthy eating, good mental health practices and other issues.

It follows, then, that finding the right balance in the relationship between the local/regional and the provincial levels can be expected to remain a persistent challenge. The infrastructure in place at the local level, the nature of the issue, and the personalities involved will all have a bearing on how the issue is addressed. The funding issue will also continue to loom large in this relationship, since in most provinces, other than Ontario, local health units receive 100 percent of their funding from the provincial level and the province will, therefore, feel justified in expecting the local or regional units to carry out its objectives. Even in Ontario, 75 percent of funding is received from the province. For their part, local public health authorities can be expected to call for higher funding levels to achieve the targets set by the province and to emphasize the importance of predictable funding levels, so they can plan for the longer term, something that will be difficult for the province to deliver. All this suggests a continuation of the push-pull dynamic between the provincial and the local/regional levels that will continue to challenge relationships in the public health area for the foreseeable future.

The intersectoral challenge

Apart from the cleavages 'between' governments, a significant dynamic also takes place 'within' governments. The *Lalonde Report* of 1974 was probably the first major government document in Canada to state that health was broader than health care, and that to have an impact on the health of the population, one needed to involve sectors outside the health field. Similarly, the *Alma Ata Declaration* of 1978, produced at the International Conference on Primary Health Care, called for "broad intersectoral collaboration" and stated that, in addition to the health sector, primary health care involved "all related sectors and aspects of national and community development, in particular agriculture, animal husbandry, food, industry, public works, communications and other sectors..." This core idea evolved into the concept of "healthy public policy," which was discussed at the first International Conference on Health Promotion in 1986, and was reflected in a consensus document, supported by the World Health Organization, called the *Ottawa Charter for Health Promotion*. The *Ottawa Charter* states that health promotion "puts health on the agenda of policy makers in all sectors and at all levels, directing them to be aware of the health consequences of their decisions and to accept their responsibilities for health" (*Ottawa Charter for Health Promotion* 1986: 2). This idea was also reflected in the same year by the Government of Canada document, *Achieving Health for All*, usually called the *Epp Report* after the Minister of Health at that time, which was tabled at the 1986 International Conference. The *Epp Report* states that "all policies, and hence all sectors, have a bearing on health," and further that "all policies which have a direct bearing on health need to be coordinated." The list of sectors needing coordination from a health perspective is acknowledged to be long, and includes such areas as income security, housing, business, agriculture, transportation and so on.

Since 1986, there has been a strong consensus in public health, in Canada and globally, about the importance of coordinating with other sectors. O'Neill et al. found a clear consensus in the literature about the necessity of inter-sectoral action to promote the health of populations (O'Neill et al. 1997: 80). More recently, the Senate Standing Committee on Social Affairs, Science and Technology stated that: "Sharing the burden of public health responsibilities across non-conventional, inter-sectoral partnerships will reinforce the public health state, especially given that 75 percent of Canadians' health is determined by physical, social and economic developments" (2002: 55).

The language around healthy public policy, which the Senate Committee reflects to some extent, has evolved into the notion of "determinants of health." Although the availability of health services is widely acknowledged as constituting one of these determinants, it is only one of many, and not necessarily the most important. No health care system, no matter how efficient and comprehensive, is able to reverse downstream impacts of public policies which are detrimental to health.

Recognizing that determinants of health usually lie outside the mandate of the health sector, Corber concludes, "To be effective in this area, public health must advocate with other sectors for healthy public policy and must develop partnerships to promote health" (Corber 2007: 38). Along these lines, Lozon and Alikhan argue in favour of "[s]haring the burden of public health responsibilities across non-conventional, inter-sectoral partnerships..." (Lozon and Alikhan 2007: 55) Yet while there is significant consensus around this point, there is little understanding about how to accomplish this objective. The literature that exists indicates that attempts to achieve inter-sectoral collaboration usually end in failure (O'Neill et al. 1997: 80). The *Epp Report* was under no illusions about the challenges inherent in this objective, stating: "It will not be an easy undertaking to coordinate policies among the various sectors, all of which obviously have their own priorities" (Epp 1986: 426).

There have been recent attempts to research the area of inter-sectoral collaboration in public health with a view of understanding better what works in this area. The WHO commissioned an analysis of 18 country case studies of health equity through inter-sectoral action in 2008 (World Health Oorganization 2008b). In addition, the Public Health Agency of Canada, in collaboration with WHO's Commission on the Social Determinants of Health, attempted to summarize what is known about inter-sectoral action in public policy, particularly as it relates to health (Public Health Agency of Canada 2007). While these works are useful as a beginning, they are just that – a beginning. Their biggest contribution at this stage may be in helping to ask the right questions rather than to provide clear answers.

Although we are situating this question in the context of public health, inter-sectoral management is not specific to this area. Indeed there is a considerable body of literature on 'horizontal management,' 'whole of government approaches,' 'joined-up government,' and other terms that have been used to describe this concept. In Canada, as in a number of countries, this has been and continues to be an elusive concept. Bakvis and Juillet have suggested that there are three types of coordination, political, policy, and administrative, and that coordination might be more readily accomplished at the administrative level than at the policy level (Bakvis and Juillet 2004). However, it is precisely at the policy level that public health seeks to work to achieve the changes needed to advance its agenda.[2]

The intragovernmental fragmentation inherent in public health may be as perplexing as the inter-governmental relations aspect. Moreover, at least one scholar has postulated that the two might be linked. Katherine Fierlbeck suggests that the lack of success that the Public Health Agency of Canada (PHAC)

---

[2] The somewhat discouraging conclusion from Bakvis and Juillet, but one with which many observers would agree, is that the Government of Canada may not have the right tools for horizontal management, and that "the organizational culture and the management frameworks are not seen as being conducive to extensive interdepartmental coordination" (2004: 47).

has had at coordinating with other federal departments has weakened its relationship with provinces and territories, and consequently weakened PHAC's coordinating capacity with provinces and territories. Fierlbeck argues that "the largest source of friction between levels of government is the lack of clear organization at the federal level" (Fierlbeck 2010: 14). This may be somewhat of an overstatement. Many of the provincial and territorial departments and agencies that form part of the Public Health Network – in other words, PHAC's interlocutors – are likely experiencing very much the same sorts of challenges within their own jurisdictions. There is no reason to expect that the inter-sectoral challenges experienced within the federal government, whether by PHAC or any other agency/department, are much different from those experienced by provincial and territorial governments, particularly the larger jurisdictions. Two cases can be referenced which attest to the challenges provincial governments face in trying to achieve inter-sectoral coordination in public health.

In the first case, British Columbia constructed a new and innovative organizational architecture around ActNowBC, its inter-sectoral health promotion strategy, precisely in order to break down the 'silos' in its own system. An inter-departmental committee was established at the assistant deputy minister level, in which ministries were expected to contribute to advance the objectives of ACTNowBC. As an incentive to encourage other ministries to participate, a fund of $15 million over three years was created from which all ministries, *other than the health ministry,* could access funds for pilot projects in support of related initiatives (British Columbia 2009: 35). The fact that the BC government found it necessary to establish a fund to encourage the participation of other departments says a great deal about the difficulty of achieving cross-departmental collaboration at the provincial level.

The second instance relates to Quebec, which is the only jurisdiction in Canada to have a legislative base to ensure inter-sectoral collaboration in public health. Section 54 of the *Public Health Act*, which was passed in 2001, mandates the minister of health to give any advice he or she considers appropriate to any other minister with respect to health promotion or initiatives having to do with the health and welfare of the population. Moreover, the same act requires that the minister of health be consulted on any legislative or regulatory measure which could impact the health of the population. In order to operationalize the latter provision, among other measures, the *Direction générale de la santé publique* has developed an intra-governmental health impact assessment mechanism with which to assess policies and initiatives of the various departments (National Collaborating Centre for Healthy Public Policy 2008: 7-8).

Both these examples suggest that provincial governments face many of the same challenges as the federal government in relation to encouraging inter-sectoral collaboration. Without going as far as Fierlbeck in seeing a one-dimensional link between inter-sectoral fragmentation at the federal level and federal/provincial/territorial friction, it is at least plausible that the two levels of fragmentation have a compounding effect on each other, thereby raising the level of complexity of finding ways to bridge the gaps.

Government-civil society relationships

The fragmentation experienced in public health does not restrict itself to the governmental sector. As discussed earlier, public health requires a societal approach. Put another way, it needs to be based on a model which acknowledges "the externalities of public health threats" (Deber et al. 2007: 69). The *Bangkok Charter* states:

> An integrated policy approach within government and international organizations, as well as a commitment to working with civil society and the private sector and across settings, are essential if progress is to be made in addressing the determinants of health (Bangkok Charter 2005: 4).

With respect to civil society, as will be discussed in chapter 6, public health is rich in the number of non-governmental and voluntary sector organizations (VSOs) that have an interest in public health generally, such as the Canadian Public Health Association; that are concerned with certain aspects of public health, such as injury prevention (Safe Communities Canada) or particular chronic or infectious diseases (Heart and Stroke Foundation of Canada, Canadian Cancer Society); or that deal with emergency response, such as the Canadian Red Cross Society. In many cases, these organizations form part of one, or more often, many consortia or networks, such as the Canadian Coalition for Public Health in the 21st century, which is composed of over 40 diverse national health associations and was formed "to provide a national forum outside government to monitor the progress of the new PHAC and provincial actions to support official public health capacity" (Chambers and Sullivan 2007: 24). The Chronic Disease Prevention Alliance of Canada was similarly formed to group together many of the organizations involved in preventing chronic diseases, such as the Canadian Cancer Society, the Heart and Stroke Foundation of Canada, and the Canadian Diabetes Association. In all, there are scores of voluntary and non-profit organizations which are involved in some way in public health.

This does not suggest that the relationship between these groups and government is always antagonistic. The core challenge is to find ways to include VSOs into the public health decision-making processes, particularly at the policy level. As chapter 6 will discuss, one can identify different types of relationships that exist between governments and voluntary sector organizations. However, as will be discussed, the relationships in place are rather limited, and, in most cases, are not particularly conducive to the development of collaborative governance.[3]

Within the broader health sector, there are also coordination challenges between the public health system and the health care system in Canada, such as hospitals, clinics, and health professionals. In 2007, McMillan and Nagpal of the Canadian Medical Association examined the state of public health infrastructure from the point of view of the front line provider, and concluded that the situation has not improved since SARS. "While some steps have been taken at the national level, there is no sense of enhanced coordination, communication or planning experienced by those professionals who desperately need support at the front line" (McMillan and Nagpal 2007: 65). The experience with the H1N1 pandemic tended to confirm this conclusion, as physicians in private practice once again complained about not being kept up to date on developments as they occurred (Interview #8: January 15, 2010).

---

[3] Of course, fragmentation also exists within the VSO community, where organizations will often compete for the 'ear' of government, and for funding, from governments as well as from private donors.

Conclusion

We have reviewed the extent to which fragmentation is a factor in public health and the challenges this represents for public health governance. To achieve the goals that public health sets for itself, following the definition offered by J.M. Last, there is a need to find ways to collaborate more effectively. This has led to frequent calls for a national public health leadership (see CIHR 2003: 38) and in some quarters to demands for the creation of a public health 'czar' in Canada (*Canadian Medical Association Journal* 2009). The parties will need to overcome the obstacles presented by a complex web of organizational autonomies and develop the mechanisms necessary to collaborate effectively toward common objectives. To use David Butler-Jones' terminology, public health will need to find a way to move from fragmentation to "alignment."

Public health, in this sense, faces an interesting quandary. On the one hand, there is general consensus that collaboration in public health is not just advisable, it is necessary (Delaney 1994: 218). The interdependence of the various actors impacting on public health makes it such that progress depends on a high level of involvement from a broad range of organizations and individuals. The forces of globalization, with the increased need to respond quickly to an increased number of public health threats, further underlines the need for a "new collaborative model" (Lozon and Alikhan 2007: 57). In spite of this, little research has been done on how to meet this challenge (Chambers and Sullivan 2007: 27). In an important essay published in 2006, Hugh Tilson and Bobbi Berkowitz acknowledge that, "[l]ittle is known about how best to organize, configure, staff, fund, and manage" the public health enterprise (Tilson and Berkowitz 2006: 909).

If fragmentation can be identified as the 'problem,' then, what is the solution? This question is not unique to public health. To a significant extent, this fragmentation, or what some have called the increasing 'turbulence' confronting policy makers, is the core issue behind the notion of modern governance (Ansell and Gash 2008: 544). Yet it may have specific meaning for the public health sector, because of its breadth. Moreover, because of the range of applications covered by public health, the answers one seeks will need to be applicable to a number of circumstances. Collaboration to improve the determinants of health, because of the long-term nature of the work, will likely be quite different from collaboration to deal with an emergency situation, such as an infectious disease outbreak. In the next chapter, we will discuss what is meant by network governance and how forms of network governance might apply to the various facets of public health.

CHAPTER 2

LOOKING AHEAD:
IS NETWORK GOVERNANCE 'THE ANSWER'?

Introduction

In the previous chapter, we discussed fragmentation in public health in Canada, and the challenges involved with coordinating the activities of a large number of organizations, governmental or otherwise, each with its own mandate, set of authorities and accountabilities and priorities, in order to achieve sought-after results. Fragmentation is not a condition that can be avoided. Rather, it is characteristic of modern society, a consequence of what one observer calls "functional and institutional specialization" (Rhodes 1997: 8). The issue is how to find a form of governance that is able to provide effective policy development and implementation in a way that would bridge rather than exacerbate societal divisions.

The challenge posed by governance in the public health area might be viewed as an example of a 'wicked problem.' Wicked problems, as a good deal of literature in the policy and management sciences has argued, are more than just complicated. They are 'wicked' because "they cannot be handled by dividing them into simple pieces in near isolation from each other" (Rittel and Webber 1973; O'Toole 1997: 46). As seen in the previous chapter, public health implicates a diverse array of actors from numerous sectors, with a wide variety of interests, thus leading to a high level of complexity in attempting to address the issues. How can these fault lines be bridged? Stated otherwise, how can one have an effective and inclusive governance regime in that sector, taking into account the level of fragmentation that characterizes the public health sector?

Network governance is a broad concept which has been conceived and applied in a variety of different ways. It is beyond the scope of this book to attempt to provide a comprehensive review of all of these formulations. Instead, in this chapter we will seek to explain how we are using the term, underline some of its key characteristics, identify its potential advantages, and discuss the applicability of network governance to public health in Canada. This will set the stage in the chapters that follow for a review, from a governance perspective, of three specific cases involving public health in Canada and what these experiences tell us about the application of this model of governance in the future.

Network governance – what is it?

The past decades have seen a veritable explosion of interest in what has come to be known as collaborative governance (see Ansell and Gash 2008: Huxham and Vangen 2005; Imperial 2005; Kamensky et al. 2004; Paquet 2011). Yet the usage of that term has varied significantly. Some scholars have used quite an expansive definition, such as in the case of Mark Imperial, who describes collaborative governance as "the means for achieving direction, control, and coordination of individuals and organizations with varying degrees of autonomy to advance joint objectives" (Imperial 2005: 282). Others have used the term in a more restrictive way (see Ansell and Gash 2008: 544). In this book, we will refer to network governance, which, depending on the definition that is used, may be seen as a somewhat narrower concept, and perhaps even a sub-set of collaborative governance. The use of this term is to underline the point that our interest is primarily in the active engagement and coordination of stakeholder organizations and networks of organizations, rather than individual citizens, or even 'clients' of the public health system. Public health is an area characterized by the presence of a large number of organized or semi-organized entities, such as governmental and non-governmental organizations, consortia, coalitions and other forms of associations. The central question we wish to ask is how to have those entities play a more effective role in the policy process, both in terms of policy development and policy implementation. Of course, network governance is a challenging concept in itself, and is open to a number of different formulations.[4] For this reason, the term requires a working definition and a brief explanation of its key characteristics as they apply to our topic.

Drawing from the definition Mandell and Steelman use for "interorganizational innovations," network governance can be defined formally as "...a spectrum of structures that involve two or more actors and may include participants from public, private, and nonprofit sectors with varying degrees of interdependence to accomplish goals that otherwise could not be accomplished independently" (Mandell and Steelman 2003: 202). The *objective* of network governance is "coordinating strategies of actors with different goals and preferences with regards to a certain problem or policy measures within an existing network of inter-organizational relations" (Kickert et al. 1997: 10).

Network governance can take quite a number of forms. It can be well-structured or less so, broad or more narrowly-based, *ad hoc* around a particular issue, or continuing. For this reason, context is of critical importance. Yet, while the concept can take shape in many different ways, the core idea behind it is that the synergy produced by the active involvement of all the relevant stakeholders in a particular area will lead to stronger policy outcomes than would have been possible if the issue had been left to only one, or a select few, actors. As Innes and Booher have observed: "There is ample evidence that such a system of distributed intelligence among linked autonomous agents can produce more desirable outcomes for a complex system at the edge of chaos than a policy devised by the most brilliant analyst or powerful bureaucrat" (Innes and Booher 2003: 48).

Without attempting to be comprehensive, three fundamental aspects of the concept are particularly germane to our discussion of how it applies to public health: the involvement of multiple and diverse actors; a non-hierarchical structure; and a mutual dependency among the actors involved. Each will be discussed in turn.

---

[4] Some authors have attempted to categorize different formulations of network governance (see Agranoff 2007; Herranz 2006).

Involvement of multiple and diverse actors

At issue here is both the *intensity* and the *scope of the interaction* between the parties. First, 'intensity' refers to a form of involvement that goes beyond simple inclusiveness or mere consultation. In network governance, participants expect that they will have a direct role in decision making as it relates to the functioning and positioning of the network, as well as the objectives it sets for itself. No large group can ever expect to function on the basis of complete consensus on all things, but network participants expect to have a process in place, even if it is loosely-structured, that involves them in decision making. In this way, networks provide a mechanism to involve a number of players in a process to resolve a policy issue or to implement a program.

With regard to scope, network governance, as a response to wicked problems, often involves stakeholders from a broad cross-section of society, including government at various levels, voluntary sector organizations and the private sector. Because of the complexity of the problems they are seeking to address, networks need to extend their reach to include various perspectives on an issue. Through the inclusion of a broad range of participants, networks seek to create a synergy that will lead to new ideas and approaches that would not have been produced, or considered, by any of the parties acting on its own (Agranoff 2007: 187). In this way, networks provide the platform "that enable the collectivity to become more than the sum of its parts..." (Posner 2009: 90).

Nonhierarchical structure

The network concept implies that the participants will not be subordinate to one another (Börzel and Panke 2007: 155). Otherwise, it would simply be a form of hierarchical/bureaucratic government. This, however, does not preclude power differentials between individuals and organizations involved in a network. Indeed, power dynamics can and do exist within networks (Kahler 2009: 13). Left unattended, these dynamics can erode the trust relations that are a necessary ingredient for the effective functioning of the network. As will be discussed in chapter 9, an important function of network leaders is to try to 'level the playing field' as much as is possible, so that the positive aspects of network governance can be realized.

The leadership function in a network may appear paradoxical, given the non-hierarchical nature of network governance. However, networks do not preclude either leadership or some degree of structure. As will be discussed, a considerable amount of attention has been given to how to 'manage' networks, referring to governance *of* networks as opposed to governance *by* networks (see Goldsmith and Eggers 2004: Huxham and Vangen 2005). Effective leadership in a network context is crucial on a number of levels. While authority is more evenly dispersed within a network than in a hierarchy, "someone still needs to come forward and help orchestrate a vision, follow through on the work plan, contact key partners, orchestrate meetings, and so on" (Agranoff 2007: 93). There will usually be one or more participants in a network, sometimes called "positional leaders," who hold more sway than others at any particular time (Huxham and Vangen 2000: 1167-1168). Often, these will be leaders not by virtue of rank in an organization, but rather more informally as a reflection of their place within a network or of personal attributes. In other words, while leadership is important in network governance, it differs from the style of leadership found in hierarchical organizations.

Finally, the issue of non-hierarchical relationships also relates to the role of governments in a network, on which more will be said below. While governments "can indirectly and imperfectly steer networks" (Rhodes 1997: 53), they will not be in a position to directly control the actions of others in a network. Very often, this steering takes "negotiation and exchange, persuasion, the forming of coalitions and strategic cooperation" (Schaap and van Twist 1997: 66). Circumstances will vary, but in general, modern governments will need to work with and within networks, and develop governing mechanisms "which do not rest on recourse to the authority and sanctions of government" (Stoker 1998: 17).

Mutual dependency of actors

Interdependence, as O'Toole's definition reflects, is also fundamental to the notion of network governance (Koppenjan and Klijn 2004: 9). The pivotal point here is that individuals and organizations recognize that they cannot accomplish their goals without the involvement of others (Kickert et al. 1997: 6). This may be due to a number of reasons relating to the need to pool resources, questions of legitimacy, access to knowledge and others. There may well be differences in the level of dependency among the various organizations. In the end, however, their inability to achieve their goals on their own remains the key incentive to participate in a network (Klijn et al. 1995: 439).

Notwithstanding the importance of interdependence, it would be naive to assume that every organization's full agenda will be completely revealed. Individuals and organizations come to the table with a set of personal or corporate objectives that they will not be inclined to share. Huxham and Vangen point out that hidden agendas are endemic to collaborations (Huxham and Vangen 2005: 81). Participants are dependent on one another to accomplish common objectives, but at the same time will often try to "steer" towards their own agenda preferences (Klijn 1997: 32; Lake and Wong 2009: 131). This can often lead to complex interactions and negotiations. However, these bargaining processes can generate policy options not previously considered and lead to policy outcomes that have a much wider basis of support than would have otherwise been the case. As Agranoff puts it: "Networks provide venues for collaboration that lead directly or indirectly to solutions" (Agranoff 2007: 173).

The need for 'entanglement strategies'

The concept of network governance becomes clearer when juxtaposed against two more conventional models of governance found in liberal democracies: the traditional/hierarchical approach and new public management (NPM). The first of these sees power concentrated in governmental structures, ordered in an hierarchical arrangement. There are other forces outside of government, of course, but government is seen as providing the leadership necessary in society. Representative institutions, such as parliaments and legislatures, supported by bureaucracies, are expected to find ways to reflect the various interests and perspectives that exist in society and find solutions to problems that arise.

As elegant and straightforward as this model may seem, the challenges of modern society has made a sole reliance on the traditional/hierarchical model untenable (Goldsmith and Eggers 2004: 180). Top-down, centralized processes are often inadequate to address complex problems, as "actors seldom have the knowledge and resources to resolve problems on their own" (Koppenjan and Klijn 2004: 8). Furthermore, measures which attempt to ignore or override some players, or restrict the ability of others to act, will often face strong resistance from actors who have an interest in the issue but who feel excluded from the process (Ibid.: 9). The end result may well lead to some form of policy paralysis, or to decisions which widen, rather than narrow, divisions within society, or to an unhappy combination of both.

Moreover, the traditional/hierarchical model represents a major loss of opportunity to harness resources that exist in society. Advances in technology and the increase in specialization have meant that knowledge is more widely distributed than in the past. Centralization often means a failure to tap the resources and potential of local actors (Kickert et al. 1997: 8).

For its part, new public management can be seen as an attempt to introduce market-like principles to the public service. Under this model, efficiency, seen as "the achievement of a supposed value for money in public services," is perceived as the overriding objective (Stoker 2006: 56). With the objective of running government like a business, this approach favours the use of private sector performance management and motivation techniques, as well as the extensive use of contracting out by governments to private sector bodies and public-private partnerships. Citizens, in this model, are often viewed as customers or clients, essentially consumers of the services governments provide.

Both the traditional/hierarchical and the NPM models reflect a need to maintain a high level of control from the centre. Under NPM, program delivery may be de-centralized from the central machinery of government, but decisions about policy are not. In addition, both models attempt to respond to the uncertainty created by a divided and differentiated policy context by reducing the number of actors involved, or limiting the roles of others, or both. Finally, neither takes sufficient account of the fact that modern society operates "in a world of networks," where accountability is much more dispersed (Rhodes 1997: 56). For these reasons, the traditional hierarchical and the NPM models, which some have categorized as "disentanglement strategies" (Koppenjan and Klijn 2004: 243) are often inadequate to deal with the challenges presented by a complex and diversified policy environment.[5]

---

[5] To be clear, we are not suggesting that network governance replaces traditional/ hierarchical and NPM in all instances. Indeed, the variety of circumstances in modern society is such that all three models co-exist in a complex environment. As Lipnack and Stamps have argued, "The age of the network includes rather than replaces its predecessors" (Lipnack and Stamps 1994: 63).

Yet what is needed in public health – and arguably, in many other domains – is not 'disentanglement' but precisely its opposite. Mechanisms are needed to bridge the fault lines described in the previous chapter, which, because of jurisdictional and other reasons, cannot be accomplished by centralizing the decision-making process and excluding parties which have a significant interest in the issue. Rather than limiting the role and the number of players, what is needed is an approach which seeks to increase the interaction between interested parties.

Weighing the costs and benefits

As much potential as network governance has in addressing complex issues of modern society, one needs to avoiding becoming, as one observer put it, "a 'cheer-leader' for unfettered cooperative public action" (O'Toole 2010: 8). In reality, the risks in network governance are undeniable (see Agranoff 2007; Koppenjan and Klijn 2004; Goldsmith and Eggers 2004; Huxham and Vangen 2005; Kickert et al. 1997). The involvement of a high number of independent organizations in the same process potentially can lead to chaos and confusion, and ultimately inaction. Such factors that could derail network governance arrangements include changes in personnel in the member organizations, changes in the priorities of the members, loss of revenue sources, and many others.

Furthermore, network governance is not cost-free. On the contrary, networks require a significant investment, particularly in time spent for the participants, if they are to succeed (Agranoff 2007: 179). Decisions and actions requiring discussion and negotiation, the communication of such, and the need to mediate differences between members are all time-intensive and resource-intensive activities. Participating in a multitude of networks simultaneously, as do many public servants and members of the voluntary and not-for-profit sectors, adds to the challenge of devoting the time and energy required to achieve positive results.

Notwithstanding the risks and costs involved in network governance, the potential benefits outweigh the disadvantages, particularly in a fragmented field such as public health. Some of the major practical benefits of network governance include:
- increased opportunities to harness resources (financial and non-financial) of other actors;

- increased opportunities for players in a broad community to learn from each other and overall to increase knowledge on a certain issue;
- increased opportunities for innovation;
- higher trust among participants, thereby enhancing social cohesion;
- greater information exchange stemming from the development of a common frame of reference; and
- improved public confidence by showing government and non-government parties working together on a specific issue.

More generally, the complexity of modern society seems to demand a more inclusive approach to governance. Agranoff, for example, suggests that, "the emerging information or knowledge era makes collaborative networking imperative" (Ibid.: 156). Similarly, in his address to the 2009 Annual Conference of the American Political Science Association, O'Toole made the point that "problems cannot be effectively addressed without drawing together organizations and actors from apparently disparate sectors and often very different levels in the governance system" (O'Toole 2010: 10). While there is a danger of over-generalizing, in many circumstances strategies of engagement are potentially more likely to lead to positive results than are strategies of disentanglement (Peters 1998: 300; Klijn et al. 1995: 452). At a minimum, such strategies can be considered successful if they promote cooperation between actors and reduce or eliminate barriers to that cooperation (Kickert et al. 1997: 175).[6]

As Kahler has pointed out: "Networks have become the intellectual centrepiece for our era" (Kahler 2009: 2). The challenge is to understand under what conditions network governance functions best and, particularly, to find the right formulation to suit the circumstances.

---

[6] There is also a strong normative element implied in the advocacy of 'entanglement strategies' in that this reflects a strong sense that liberal democracies *ought* to provide their citizens with a greater opportunity to become players in the public policy process beyond simply exercising (or not exercising) their right to vote every few years. Networks, therefore, may be key to a redefinition of liberal democracy (see Box et al. 2001; Stoker 2006).

Conclusion: Applying network governance to public health

Given the above, it would seem that public health is ideally suited for network governance approaches. First, to achieve the results it sets for itself, public health must find ways of bridging the fault lines discussed in the previous chapter. Second, the sector is populated by innumerable governmental and non-governmental organizations and coalitions which are actively involved in the area in some capacity. This, therefore, creates a need for some level of coordination to maximize the benefit of the knowledge and the resources, material and non-material, that the various players contribute to the field. Furthermore, working through networks provides a vehicle to reach and engage at the community level, which is of crucial importance if public health interventions are to be successful.

At the global level, public health advocates have been calling for a more inclusive and expansive approach to public health since the 1970s and 1980s. In fact, this is a central part of what is often called "New Public Health." The charter produced at the first international conference on health promotion – known as the *Ottawa Charter* – states that health promotion "demands coordinated action by all concerned: by governments, by health and other social and economic sectors, by nongovernmental and voluntary organization [sic], by local authorities, by industry and by the media" (*Ottawa Charter* 1986). The same perspective is reflected more recently in The World Health Organization-sponsored *Bangkok Charter for Health Promotion,* which points out that: "Partnerships, alliances, networks and collaborations provide exciting and rewarding ways of bringing people and organizations together around common goals and joint actions to improve the health of populations" (*Bangkok Charter* 2005).

In Canada, as cited earlier, the importance of working through networks was explicitly endorsed by the Chief Public Health Officer of Canada in his first report. Yet there is much to be learned about how the network approach can and should be applied to the various circumstances of public health. As mentioned earlier, the application of network governance is highly contextual, and applications need to suit the particular circumstances to which they relate. For example, health promotion and chronic disease prevention exercises, which inevitably require broad horizontal, multi-stakeholder approaches, will have significantly different governance requirements compared to governance in the context of public health emergencies, such as in the case of a pandemic. It is of course not possible to review all such circumstances in this book. However, in the next three chapters, we will examine governance in the context of three specific 'theatres' involving public health in Canada: the Pan-Canadian Public Health Network (PNH), the emergency preparedness and response context, particularly as seen in the SARS crisis of 2003 and the H1N1 pandemic of 2009, and the Canadian Heart Health Initiative (CHHI). In each case, one can argue that the model that was employed, as in the cases of the PHN and CHHI, or that was advocated in much of the post-crisis literature about SARS, was inadequately conceptualized or applied from a network governance perspective. All of these pose particular challenges and necessitate applying distinct strategies. However, it is by examining specific cases such as these that one can learn more about how network governance can be applied in future public health initiatives.

II – PUBLIC HEALTH GOVERNANCE IN CANADA: THREE THEATRES

CHAPTER 3

GOVERNANCE AND
THE PUBLIC HEALTH NETWORK:
TOO MUCH OR NOT ENOUGH?

Introduction

The Pan-Canadian Public Health Network (PHN) is the centrepiece of public health governance at the national level. It represents a deliberate attempt to build in a strong element of collaboration in its workings, in large part motivated by the breakdowns that occurred during the SARS crisis of 2003. As its name implies, the concept of network was key to how this collaboration was to be operationalized. However, as will be discussed in this chapter, the model, as originally established in 2005, while representing a significant departure from previous practices, falls short of a network governance perspective in a number of significant ways. Furthermore, we will argue that the 2011 changes represent a shift towards a less flexible, more vertically integrated structure, and hence constitutes a step away from the notion of network governance. Overall, the argument that will be presented in this chapter is that while the PHN reflects a recognition of the importance of collaboration and working through networks, it is an inadequate response to the challenges of working in a fragmented policy environment.

The Pan-Canadian Public Health Network (2005 edition)

The PHN was established in 2005, and underwent a substantial review in 2009-11, which has led to significant changes in structure. For the student of network governance, it is important to follow the changes in structure and the rationale given for making them. For this reason, we will begin by discussing the PHN from its inception until the latter part of 2010. Following this, we will review the changes to the structure approved in 2011 and discuss what they mean for the potential to realize network governance in the public health sector.

As stated above, to a large extent, the PHN was established in the wake of the SARS crisis of 2003. (Chapter 4 reviews the major events surrounding the SARS crisis.) A broad consensus emerged that the response to the SARS events revealed the weak and disorganized state of public health in Canada, and that a major cause of this was the failure among the governments in particular to collaborate with each other. The National Advisory Committee on SARS and Pubic Health stated categorically that "the single largest impediment to dealing successfully with future public health crises is the lack of a collaborative framework and ethos among different levels of government" (*Naylor Report* 2003: 212). The PHN was a response to this call for greater collaboration in that it was meant to correct the breakdowns that appeared during the SARS crisis.

A secondary, but still important trigger for the establishment of the PHN was the perceived need to bring some order to the various collaborative bodies that preceded the PHN, many of which had been in existence for some time. *Partners in Public Health*, a report of the federal/provincial/territorial Special Task Force on Public Health, which served as the guiding document for the creation of the PHN, states that the PHN was meant to correct "the public health experience of *ad hoc*, uncoordinated, collaboration on public health issues, often through numerous one-off committees, task forces, and functions" (*Partners in Public Health* 2005: 3). As part of its review, the task force documented 84 federal/provincial/territorial committees with roles and mandates related to public health (Ibid.: 39).

The PHN was envisioned "as the primary vehicle for multilateral sharing and exchange between federal, provincial and territorial public health institutions and professionals" (Ibid.: 3). The *Partners* document makes clear that this was meant as a forum for information and knowledge sharing, not for joint decision making. The point is made more than once that the PHN is to provide "a mechanism for intergovernmental collaboration and coordination on public health issues *while respecting the authority and jurisdiction of each government to manage public health operations within its own domain*" (Ibid.: 20, emphasis added). Moreover, it is reflective of the role of the PHN as a technical knowledge and information sharing body, that membership on the council is expected to consist of "senior officials...who have technical knowledge of public health..." (Ibid.: 21).

The structure of the PHN is illustrated in Figure 1. At the head of the structure is the PHN Council. It is co-chaired by the Chief Public Health Officer for Canada (CPHO) and one of the provincial/territorial members on a rotating basis. Provincial/territorial members are represented by a senior official, often a chief medical officer of health, or an assistant deputy minister (ADM) level representative. The ADM from the First Nations and Inuit Branch of Health Canada is also included to address the circumstances of First Nations people on reserve and Inuit people. It is clear that the council was deliberately structured as an inter-governmental body. The *Partners* document indicates that non-government organizations can be invited, as appropriate, "to participate and help inform Council decisions on issues that are directly relevant to their mandate or expertise" (Ibid.: 27). They are not, however, to be regular members of the PHN Council, nor are they expected to participate as decision makers. Furthermore, they participate by invitation only, and are there to provide technical information, not to represent a particular organization or sector.

FIGURE 1: Structure of The PHN (2005 edition)

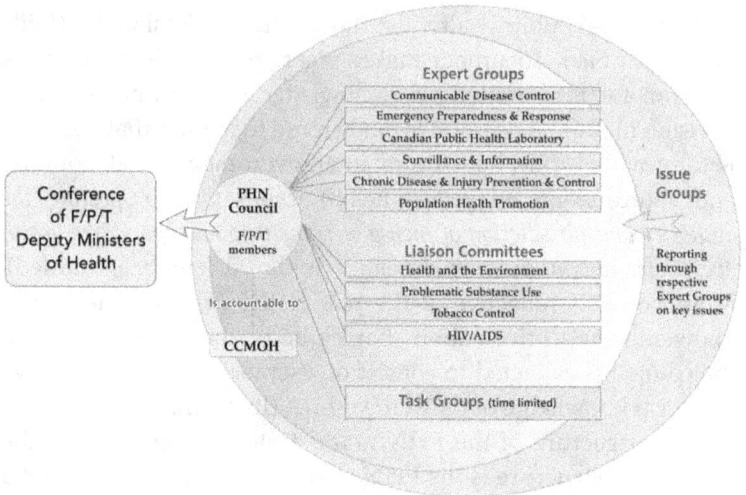

Source: Pan-Canadian Public Health Network. 2011. Annual Report 2010-2011, *Ottawa: Public Health Agency of Canada, page 7. Reprinted with permission.*

As seen in Figure 1, the council reports to the federal/provincial/territorial Conference of Deputy Ministers of Health (CDMH), which sets the PHN's priorities and directs their work. "It is the CDMH which will identify the scope of the mandate of the Network and will hold the members on the Council accountable for the deliverables and performance of the Network" (Ibid.: 21). The CDMH, in turn, reports to the Conference of Ministers of Health.

Reporting to the PHN Council are six 'expert groups,' the terminology used again reinforcing the point that these are meant to be composed of individuals with technical expertise, rather than decision makers. They are responsible for the following areas: communicable disease; emergency preparedness and response; laboratories; surveillance and information; non-communicable (chronic) disease and injury prevention and control; and population health promotion.

Each of the expert groups is co-chaired by a federal representative, usually at the director general level, and a provincial/territorial representative on a rotating basis.[7]

---

[7] This author was the federal co-chair for the Population Health Promotion Expert Group from 2005 to 2008.

Apart from the governmental representatives, there may be representation from university researchers or from others with specialized knowledge in the area. The PHN Council provides direction to these groups about priorities, as well as approving their work plans, and generally monitoring their progress.

At the next level are issue groups, which are assigned a specific issue to deal with. For the most part they are co-chaired in a similar way to expert groups, although there are instances, as with the case of the Healthy Living Issue Group, where there is a third co-chair to represent voluntary sector organizations (VSOs). Their work is overseen by the relevant expert group.

Below this level is a myriad of work groups, task groups, and sub-groups established to look at specific questions. They can be both *ad hoc* or continuing. Their membership will be federal, provincial and territorial officials, and can involve others, but will often be less formally structured than expert or issue groups. Finally, as mentioned above, there is a set of what are known as 'liaison committees,' such as those on nutrition and health and the environment, which address public health issues but which function outside the 'orbit' of the PHAC.

An important component of the PHN is the Council of Chief Medical Officers of Health. This body, which pre-dates the PHN, is exclusively composed of physicians. It is co-chaired by the same individuals as the PHN Council, and has a high degree of overlapping memberships with that body. The *Operational Review* conducted on the PHN cites that, at the time of writing (September 2010), 9 of the 18 members of the PHN Council members also sat on the CCMOH, although these numbers can fluctuate (Pan-Canadian Public Health Network 2010a: 12). This is not a coincidence. *Partners in Public Health*, without being directive, states that there would be substantial benefits "if the Council's membership mirrors the existing Council of Chief Medical Officers of Health" (*Partners in Public Health* 2005: 21). Although it is positioned somewhat outside the PHN hierarchy of committees, as can be seen from Figure 2 (page 60), it functions as a 'community of practice' and is influential in providing technical expertise to the PHN Council and playing an advocacy role within the PHN (Interview #1: May 9, 2011).

The PHN (2005): A breakthrough towards network governance?

The PHN will be discussed using three criteria: structural flexibility, inclusiveness, and lateral 'reach'. With regard to the first, the literature on network governance emphasizes the importance of flexible structures to allow for ideas and creativity to flow smoothly within a network (see Kickert et al. 1997: 10). Secondly, inclusiveness is fundamental to network governance since bridging divisions in society implies an ability to include participants from a cross-section of that society, particularly governments, civil society, and the private sector. Finally, lateral reach refers to the ability to open and maintain a dialogue with other policy sectors, which, as discussed in chapter 1, is necessary for public health to be able to reach its objectives. It has also been referred to as inter-sectoral collaboration, horizontal management, and joined-up government.

Structural flexibility

The names used to describe the various components, expert groups, issue groups etc., reflect an attempt to underline the collaborative aspect of the process, largely built on the notion of knowledge, whether existing, sharing or building, rather than revolving around the roles of individuals representing the interests of their respective governments. The member of the Communicable Disease Expert Group from a specific province, say Saskatchewan, without compromising the positions of his jurisdiction, is there primarily to contribute to the fight against communicable disease. Although not explicitly stated, one infers from *Partners in Public Health* that the thinking behind the PHN was that a common search for responses to public health challenges would overshadow jurisdictional differences and facilitate collaboration and cooperation. In it, the PHN is described as "a voluntary association and cooperation [sic] whose efforts to collaborate are to enhance public health across the country" (*Partners in Public Health* 2005: 21).

Viewed from the perspective of intensity, the PHN is quite impressive. Through its elaborate and complex tapestry of formal and informal network structures, it reflects a level of commitment to the value of collaboration. Yet from the perspective of network governance, the PHN may not represent as radical a departure from the more traditional federal/provincial/territorial structures as might appear on the surface. The nomenclature of the various groups in the PHN is novel, but the structure and functioning of these committees does not appear to be qualitatively different from the federal/provincial/territorial committee structure that existed in Health Canada before the SARS crisis and the creation of the Public Health Agency of Canada. Prior to 2005, the ADM of the Population and Public Health Branch, as it was then, co-chaired the Advisory Committee on Public Health and Health Security which resembled the PHN in many respects. It is arguable that what differentiates the PHN groups is a stronger than usual culture of collaboration, perhaps owing to the origins of the Network. The importance of collaboration is a recurring theme – perhaps *the* recurring theme – in the *Naylor Report*. Likewise, in the opening sentence of their transmission letter to ministers of health for *Partners in Public Health*, the co-chairs of the special task force responsible for the document, Dr. Perry Kendall and Ian Shugart, remind ministers of their decision in the aftermath of the SARS events "to chart a course for greater collaboration in public health" (*Partners in Public Health* 2005).

The effort to overcome jurisdictional differences by emphasizing the knowledge aspect component of the work is consistent with attempts to build a collaborative style of operations. For the most part, however, these groups operate as intergovernmental committees, with the addition of a limited number of university researchers and other non-governmental bodies with relatively ambiguous roles. Furthermore, the fact that the PHN reports to a senior-level intergovernmental committee, the Conference on Deputy Ministers of Health, necessarily limits how far the PHN can depart from a more orthodox model of governance. As will be discussed below, the 2011 revisions not only confirm this tendency, but indeed have shifted the balance in favour of a more hierarchical approach.

A second factor which potentially limits the ability of the PHN to be innovative is the lack of distinction between the different types of networks which are encompassed within the PHN. The point has been made that network governance operates "in the shadow of bureaucracy" (Scharf 1994: 37). There is no set 'sweet spot' of where vertical authority intersects with horizontal governance for maximum results. This will vary according to circumstances and the type of network involved. Finding the appropriate balance between the layers of horizontal and vertical governance is a key challenge, perhaps *the* key challenge of modern governance. The 'ideal' combination needs to suit the particular context in which it operates.

The PHN, however, is not one monolithic network but rather encompasses many different types of networks, with a significant variation of stated purpose and objectives. The PHN networks could be placed at different points along a continuum, based on their level of centralization or decentralization. In some cases, such as in the area of emergency preparedness and response, the objective is to achieve an 'action' network, with defined roles for various players. This can be seen in the recommendations in *Partners for Public Health* for a formal federal/provincial/territorial agreement, to be called an Agreement on Mutual Aid During an Emergency, with a higher level of centralization than what one might see in other areas (*Partners in Public Health* 2005: 12). While *Partners* did not provide details about what this agreement should contain, it is designed to lead to concrete action and joint decision making. Another recommendation along similar lines is for the development of federal, provincial, territorial data sharing agreements and corresponding enabling regulations and legislation (Ibid.: 11-12).

Networks in the area of health promotion and chronic disease prevention, on the other hand, reflect quite a different model.[8] While the participants share common objectives, follow-up action is left to the discretion of the respective jurisdiction. In these cases, members of the expert groups will work together on knowledge products, such as studies or reports, but joint action on the basis of these products is neither requested nor expected. The fact that the PHN houses different types of networks is not, in itself, problematic; indeed, it is highly advisable that it should do so, given the wide range of circumstances in public health. What is of concern is the lack of a clear differentiation between types of networks, and therefore the lack of an explicit recognition that each may need to function differently – with different types of competencies, relationships, and accountabilities – to achieve its objectives.

[8] Networks have been categorized in a number of ways. A particularly useful categorization is found in Agranoff (2007: 10), who proposes four types of networks: action, outreach, developmental and informational. Examples of each of these can be found in public health in Canada.

Notwithstanding the above, expert groups under the original manifestation of the PHN enjoyed a fair amount of flexibility to act as they saw fit. Although workplans were required and submitted to the PHN Council for approval, the level of oversight was relatively light. To a significant extent, expert groups were free to set many of their own priorities, and to develop outside partnerships they considered appropriate. According to the operational review, some participants saw this as problematic, and expressed concern that expert groups were allowed too much autonomy and developed a tendency to 'do their own thing.' As will be discussed below, this was one of the perceived flaws in the PHN that the operational review, in its final recommendations, attempted to correct.

In the end, while it fell short in the areas noted above, the PHN as it was originally constructed was a step toward a less hierarchical, more flexible style of governance from the perspective of network governance. As we will see below, however, many of the more flexible aspects that characterized the original PHN are to be dismantled, or at least modified, by the 'new' PHN in the interests of greater efficiency and smoother operations.

Inclusiveness

Although *Partners in Public Health* states that "it will be important for the Network to include the participation of non-governmental organizations (NGOs) with public health expertise, capacity and interest" (Ibid.:19), civil society and, in particular, voluntary sector organizations (VSOs) form only a marginal place in the PHN structure. This is not to deny the relationships between public health VSOs and either the PHAC or Health Canada. As chapter 6 will illustrate, there is a great deal of interaction in public health with VSOs. The point remains, however, that the role of the VSOs in the PHN, as the pre-eminent network structure at the national level, is quite weak, particularly from a policy perspective. To the extent that VSOs have been included in the PHN, it is primarily for their technical expertise, rather than for the broader perspectives they might offer on behalf of the constituencies they represent. McMillan and Nagpal have pointed out that while the Network is a good mechanism for intergovernmental coordination, "[t]he ability for other stakeholders to contribute and obtain information remains limited and unsatisfactory" (McMillan and Nagpal 2007: 64).

Secondly, *Partners in Public Health* states that "the building of a new structure for public health partnerships is also an opportunity to determine how best to include Aboriginal Peoples" (*Partners in Public Health* 2005: 19). Unfortunately, although attempts have been made, this is a recommendation that has not been acted upon five years after the establishment of the PHN. As it stands, there are no representatives of the National Aboriginal Organizations on either the council or in the expert groups. The Healthy Living Issue Group includes a representative for each of the Aboriginal peoples – First Nations, Métis and Inuit – but is one of the few, if not the only, committee within the PHN to have done so. At the council level, the ADM of the First Nations and Inuit Branch of Health Canada has been invited as a regular participant to provide a perspective from that sector, but this person is obviously not in a position to represent the views of Aboriginal peoples. There was also an Aboriginal person on the PHN Council from 2005 to 2008, but this individual made clear that she participated on her own behalf, not as a representative of any Aboriginal organization or group. The lack of Aboriginal representation on the PHN became publicly debated around the H1N1 events of 2009. Several of the Aboriginal leaders made the point that the lack of Aboriginal representation exacerbated the pandemic, and may have led to a higher level of mortality and morbidity in some regions, such as northern Manitoba (Webster 2009). Whether or not this can accurately be stated, it is evident that First Nations, Métis and Inuit have very distinct public health challenges and that attempts to address them will require the direct involvement of their representatives.

Lateral reach

The PHN may be seen as an 'epistemic community,' which can be defined as a network of professionals with recognized expertise and competence in a particular domain and an authoritative claim to policy-relevant knowledge within that domain or issue area" (Haas 1992: 3). The question is whether the existence of an epistemic community, in itself, limits the ability of such a community to reach other policy communities because of the extent to which its members will have a shared set of normative beliefs: shared causal beliefs, shared notions of validity, and a common policy enterprise. The field of public health is one obviously dominated by health professionals, primarily physicians who have a public health background. The *Public Health Agency of Canada Act* stipulates that the person holding the office of the Chief Public Health Officer "shall be a health professional who has qualifications in the field of public health" (*Public Health Agency of Canada Act* 2006). Similar stipulations exist regarding the positions of the medical officers of health at the provincial/territorial level. We have already noted the influential role that the Council of Chief Medical Officers of Health has in the PHN, and the fact that, at present, a major portion of the PHN Council is composed of members who also sit on the CCMOH. The leadership provided by the PHN Council and the CCMOH will naturally infuse throughout the PHN, and will be reinforced by the fact that many (though not all) of the leadership positions in the various expert groups and issue groups will be taken by individuals with backgrounds as health professionals.

The fact that members of an epistemic communities share a common perspective, in a sense a common 'language,' can often facilitate arriving at a general consensus among the participants of that community. In the case of public health, the participants will tend to see themselves as allies to advance a public health agenda within their respective governments, as the case study of the Canadian Heart Health Strategy (chapter 5) suggests. Rather than developing adversarial relationships, they, in fact, become advocates for a common 'cause.'

At the same time, however, as Peters has observed, the existence of an epistemic community, while it promotes internal consensus, "makes it less likely that they will be able to deal effectively with other groups who lack the common perspective on the issues" (Peters 2007: 72). Having a common language and perspective would likely be very helpful when attempting to contain an infectious disease outbreak. One would expect fairly easy agreement on the threat to the public posed by the disease and on the measures needed to deal with it. The recent experience with H1N1 generally supports this proposition, as there were few differences – although there were some vocal dissenters – between the medical officers of health in each of the jurisdictions over how to respond to the disease.

A different dynamic, however, takes place to deal with the longer term objectives of public health, such as the encouragement of health promoting public policies. In these cases, leaders in the public health community must deal with representatives of other sectors who do not necessarily have the same training or share the same language or perspective. The ability to talk across different policy communities is never easy. Much has been made in public management of the existence of policy 'silos' and the need to break through those silos (see, for example, Peters 1998). The point to be made here is not that public health professionals cannot or will not cross these boundaries, but that belonging to an epistemic community can make it more difficult to move outside those boundaries to engage others in policy sectors that have an important impact on the health of the population.

Perhaps related to the above, relatively weak intersectoral mechanisms were established to deal with issues pertaining to public health. The network infrastructure described above is impressive at bringing together public servants from federal/provincial/territorial jurisdictions working in the area of public health. However, it reveals little in the way of mechanisms to deal with other policy sectors.

The lack of intersectoral mechanisms at the national level is not a trivial matter. Whole of government approaches are regularly cited as being necessary to achieve the more fundamental aspects of the public health agenda (see, for example, the *Ottawa Charter* 1986; the *Bangkok Charter* 2005; and World Health Organization 2008a) Many of the broader issues affecting health are at play at the national level, and the lack of effective mechanisms at this level, at least as they relate to the PHN, are detrimental to achieving the longer-range aspirations of public health.

Although the PHN has reached out to some other policy sectors, such as the abovementioned federal/provincial/territorial Committee on Health and Environment, there are few such examples. For the most part the PHN operates in the public health policy 'bubble.'

The 2011 Operational Review

Beginning in the fall of 2009 to the end of 2010, the PHN underwent a review of its operations. A consulting firm was hired to study what had been accomplished since the establishment of the PHN in 2005, to survey extensively the views of the participants in the process about their level of satisfaction in the network, and to suggest what might be done to improve its functioning. As part of the exercise, the Pan-Canadian Public Health Network Operational Review Project was asked to look further into the recommendations made in an earlier (2008) review of the PHN. The 2008 review had been carried out at the instigation of the Conference of Deputy Ministers of Health, who had expressed issues and concerns in three areas:

- strengthening communications and accountability;
- the structure and management of the PHN; and
- federal/provincial/territorial relations.

The final report was submitted in September 2010, with 33 recommendations "to strengthen the PHN and position the Network to meet its mandate and future challenges within public health for Canada" (Pan-Canadian Public Health Network 2010a: 3).

The report begins with a general statement of satisfaction that overall, the PHN is seen by the participants as being successful in carrying out its mandate, and that it had had a positive impact in improving the level of collaboration across jurisdictions. At the same time, the report states that "a vast majority" of those surveyed had identified several challenges faced by the PHN, and felt that there was a need to review its operations.

The areas identified in the report are quite wide-ranging and cover the areas of mandate, structures and accountability, roles and representation, resources/supports, management support, planning and priorities, decision making and partnerships. It also proposes a revised organizational chart, presented as Figure 2, which was approved by the Conference of Deputy Ministers of Health in December 2010. For our purposes, a number of areas are particularly relevant.

FIGURE 2: Structure of The PHN (2011 edition)

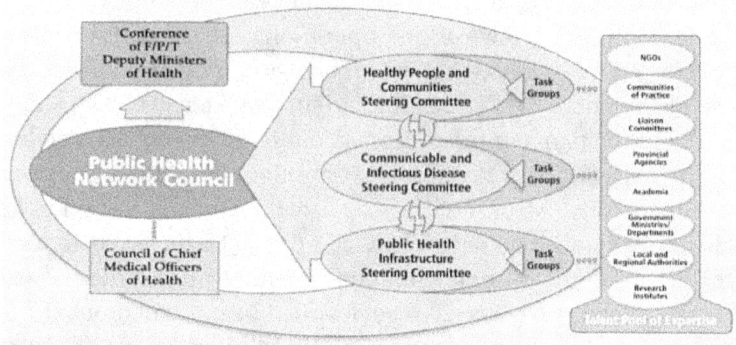

Source: Pan-Canadian Public Health Network. 2011. Annual Report 2010-2011, *Ottawa: Public Health Agency of Canada, page 10. Reprinted with permission.*

More structure, less flexibility

To begin with, the report represents an interesting shift from the original positioning around the question of representation. Whereas *Partners in Public Health* suggested a strategy of overcoming, or perhaps sidelining, jurisdictional issues by focusing on knowledge and expertise, the review puts jurisdictional representation back into prominence. The expert groups, which, significantly, are now called "Steering Committees," are directed to put federal/provincial/territorial representation as a 'first priority,' with technical expertise as 'a secondary asset.' This change in 'labeling' addresses the ambiguity around whether a participant was there because of her/his substantive expertise or as a representative of a government, a concern that was raised in the consultations. It is also meant to reflect the reality that many who were sitting on the expert groups were not subject experts. With the changes to the PHN, responsibility for dealing with technical public health issues are assigned to task groups, which are formed for specific, time-limited purposes, and whose work is mandated and overseen by one of four steering committees.[9]

Second, the final report of the PHN Operational Review conveys a clear sense that the process needs to be centralized and

[9] The Conference of Deputy Ministers of Health has decided, for the time being, not to operationalize one of the four steering committees. The issues that were to be addressed by the Steering Committee on Environmental Health and Safety will be dealt with by the PHN Council (Interview #56: September 28, 2011).

streamlined so that it can achieve its objectives more efficiently and effectively (Ibid.: 6). In this light, a number of measures were proposed to 'tighten up' the process, in other words, to increase the level of top-down vertical integration. The key step in this direction is to ensure that all work undertaken by the network is in conformity with the strategic directions and priorities, as set by the PHN Council. The steering committees are to ensure alignment with priorities, and also to see that the work is done "while applying a task-based, project management approach" (Ibid.).

From an organizational standpoint, a number of measures reflect a more centralized approach. Starting from the top, there will be quarterly reporting to federal/provincial/territorial deputy ministers about priorities, objectives, deliverables and timelines. The process of developing – and defending – these quarterly reports will then put the PHN Council in position to "routinely track the status of the work plans and deliverables of each of the groups mandated by Council" (Ibid.: 26). A new "Committee of co-chairs" will be created, composed of the PHN Council Executive and the co-chairs of each of the steering committees "to effectively manage the work and results of the PHN" (Ibid.: 32). The provincial/territorial co-chairs of the steering committees, where possible, are to be drawn from members on the PHN Council, in order to ensure that the council's intentions are understood and carried out (Ibid.: 32). Formal budget allocations will be made to each steering committee and task group based on pre-approved work plans and objectives, and based on the business planning cycle. Performance agreements will also be prepared for co-chairs and group members. Finally, the Network Secretariat, which is being strengthened to provide enhanced administrative, policy support and process facilitation skills, will report directly to the PHN Council so that it "can be better able to direct the activities of the Secretariats" (Ibid.). As a part of this, the PHN will strengthen its capacity for accountability, project management, strategic alignment, and business and work planning.

No change is proposed regarding the role of the Council of Chief Medical Officers of Health. It was felt that the CCMOH should continue to function as a separate structure so that it could provide technical expertise and continue to provide its advocacy function (Ibid.: 37). Somewhat surprisingly, the final report warns against potential duplication and inefficiencies resulting from overlaps in membership between the Council and the CCMOH, but makes no recommendation on how to resolve this.

More limited inclusion

The 2011 changes also touch on how the PHN relates to groups outside the government sector. As stated above, the PHN Council and the steering committees – the strategic committees of the PHN – would be clearly established as intergovernmental committees, with members representing their jurisdiction as a first priority (Ibid.: 2). The final report recognizes that the PHN needs to work more closely with VSOs, universities, provincial agencies, and others. However, as Figure 2 on page 60 indicates, these groups would be asked to participate as part of a task group, rather than as part of a steering committee. It would also be clear that they participate on the basis of their expertise, and not to represent an organization or a policy interest. Moreover, there would be no continuing relationship with these groups, as they would be disbanded when the particular task in which they were involved has been accomplished.[10]

The role in the PHN with regard to Aboriginal groups is left more ambiguous, in spite of the fact that this issue has been outstanding since the initiation of the PHN in 2005. While Aboriginal 'engagement' is sought, there is no provision to include national Aboriginal organizations into the PHN structure at this stage. Instead, another group, the National Collaborating Centre on Aboriginal Health, is asked to develop recommendations on the best way "to formally integrate Aboriginal health into the work of PHN Steering Committees" (Ibid.: 4). One possibility being considered is to have an advisor on Aboriginal health sit on the PHN to provide expertise in the area, but not to represent the policy views of Aboriginal peoples. This would be established on a one-year basis, and seen as a possible first step in engaging Aboriginal peoples more directly into the PHN process (Interview #56: September 28, 2011).

Minor changes in lateral reach

The operational review did not recommend significant changes that would improve the ability of the PHN to reach

---

[10] The possibility of maintaining these groups in some capacity, perhaps as virtually 'communities of practice,' was under discussion at the time of writing (Interview #56: September 28, 2011).

other policy sectors more effectively. Since the approval of the recommendations, however, the CDMH directed the PHN council to "explore collaboration" with the forum of federal/provincial/territorial ministers of Sport, Physical Activity, and Recreation (SPAR), as well as provincial/territorial ministers of Education related to the childhood obesity issue, and specifically to discuss the after-school time period (Interview #54: July 7, 2011). However, the relationship with ministers of SPAR is not a long reach, as the federal minister of health has been a member of this committee for many years, as have some of the provincial and territorial health and/or health promotion ministers. Furthermore, the issue on which they will consider collaborating, while important, is relatively narrow and presumably time-limited.

Apart from the above steps, which remain relatively modest, the revised PHN structure does not suggest much improvement in the horizontal reach of that network. Indeed, the final result may be in the opposite direction, in the sense that the 'tighter' management structure and operating framework could make it more difficult for the new steering committees to engage with other sectors if such engagement requires an investment of time and resources, as it usually does.

The PHN (2011 edition): Increased efficiency, but at what price?

While the PHN Operational Review and the recommendations made in the final report were seen as a series of steps to streamline the PHN's operations, rather than a radical departure from the original PHN structure, they represent an important turning point for the network. Viewed against our discussion of the PHN in its initial incarnation, the changes seek to address some important issues. In the first place, steps have been taken to include in the PHN at least some of the public health issues in which Health Canada has the federal lead. For example, the environmental health and safety issue will now be dealt with by the PHN Council, although the steering committee on that subject recommended in the operational review will not be established for the time being (Interview #56: September 28, 2011). Previously, this issue existed only on the periphery of the PHN.

Furthermore, the final report recommends enhanced linkages between the council and the liaison committees, such as those on problematic substance use and HIV/AIDS (Pan-Canadian Public Health Network 2010b: 6).[11] Second, there is, in the treatment of the emergency response, a tacit acknowledgement that the PHN contains different types of networks which need to be seen and treated differently. A distinction was made between 'peace time' structures of the PHN and those that would be put in place in emergency situations. A process was established to look at this issue in more detail and make recommendations. While this falls short of a careful assessment of all networks under the PHN, it implicitly acknowledges that a 'one-size-fits-all' approach is not appropriate for public health networks. Third, measures were taken to strengthen the capacity and competencies of the PHN Secretariat in areas such as coordination and facilitation, although these seem to have been put forward primarily in the context of business planning and reporting cycles.

Taken together, however, the recommendations point to a shift in the balance between the horizontal and vertical axes of governance in the direction of a greater level of top-down control over the operations of the network. The federal/provincial/territorial deputy ministers have more opportunities to monitor the work that the PHN is undertaking. The PHN Council, in turn, through strategic planning instruments as well as organizational measures, is in greater control of the activities taking place within the network. The steering committees, through business cycle plans, work plans and budgeting measures, are in a much better position to control the task groups, which, in any event, are to be disbanded once their assignment has been completed.

It is difficult to argue with the objective of seeking greater efficiencies in the process, and ensuring that accountabilities are defined for activities that take place within the network. Of greater concern is the fact that the scope of the PHN seems to have narrowed somewhat as a result. More open discussions with individuals and groups outside of government may still happen in other venues, but are less likely to occur within the PHN than was previously the case. The involvement of

[11] On the other hand, no steps appear to have been taken to integrate nutrition more closely in the PHN.

outside parties, which was not strong in the original PHN, has been significantly weakened as a result of the changes. While it is premature to arrive at any firm conclusions, since the changes are being implemented at the time of writing and it still remains to be seen what effect they will have in practice, the possibility remains that some opportunities for innovation and creativity may be lost as the price to be paid for this increased level of vertical control. Admittedly, the report acknowledges that the PHN "supports significant work and progress in public health that may not need to hit the DMs' table." However, this observation seems incongruous with the overall thrust of the report, and is not reflected in any of the specific recommendations made. Furthermore, there is evidence in at least one area, emergency preparedness and response, that networks which existed under the previous PHN structure, such as the Council of Emergency Social Services Directors, have been left out of the new PHN and are, in a sense, 'orphaned' (Interview #55: July 14, 2011).

The increased emphasis on jurisdictional representation within the PHN appears to point in the same direction. The risk is that the clearer role definition around jurisdiction will discourage more open discussions and creative thinking than was the case under the original incarnation of the network. While the original vision provided by the authors of *Partners in Public Health* may have introduced a level of ambiguity in the roles of the players, the focus on expertise as a way to overcome jurisdictional disagreements encouraged a level of thinking outside the box. A stronger focus on jurisdictional representation suggests a return to a more conventional approach.

As noted earlier, the original (2005) manifestation of the PHN contained important deficiencies from a network governance perspective. Still, it represented a different approach to the involvement of federal/provincial/territorial governments, supplemented with a modest level of participation from the voluntary sector community. Unfortunately, the 2011 changes left unattended some of the important deficiencies, while introducing changes that might remove some of the flexibility from the operations of the network. As a result, the changes to the PHN could represent a move towards smoother, efficient operations, at the expense of a more inclusive and dynamic process.

Conclusion

This discussion of the public health network infrastructure must be kept in perspective. Public health as a sector may well have been more proactive than many other public policy sectors in attempting to build collaborative mechanisms. The *Naylor Report* and *Partners in Public Health* are both remarkable documents in their appreciation of the importance of working collaboratively. The attempts to implement their recommendations, in spite of some shortcomings, represent a rather courageous effort to develop further the collaborative aspects of public health.

The evolution of the PHN seems to reflect the interplay between the horizontal and the vertical forces, and the efforts to find the 'right' balance between the two. While the initial construct of this network reflected a strong appreciation on the importance of collaboration, the 2011 changes seems to reflect a desire to reassert a stronger level of top-down control of the process and to strengthen the role of the PHN as an intergovernmental structure, rather than as a forum that would include broader societal elements. It may well be that the shorter term, more operational aspects of public health, such as those related to responses to infectious disease outbreaks, may function more efficiently. On the other hand, the structure, as designed, does not seem suited to including other policy sectors, or civil society, to help address the longer term issues facing public health, specifically those relating to disease prevention and health promotion.

To our question about whether the public health infra-structure, as see through the PHN, is too much or not enough to deal effectively with the modern challenges of public health, the answer is probably 'both.' It is 'too much' in the sense that the (increasing) level of vertical control may have a tendency to discourage more creative approaches from percolating up the chain. At the same time, it is 'too little' in the sense that it fails to fully engage those outside the public health intergovernmental circle, such as civil society, members of other policy communities, and Aboriginal organizations. It may be as one key informant suggested, that these elements can be accommodated through other mechanisms, rather than expecting the PHN to be the centrepiece for all relationships affecting public health (Interview #1: May 9, 2011). However, as chapter 6 will discuss, there is as yet no formal mechanism, or even a framework, for dealings with the voluntary sector. The same can be said in reference to relationships with First Nations, Inuit and Métis peoples.

There is, unfortunately, no simple formula that can be used to address the deficiencies that have been raised. Nevertheless, the literature on network governance offers a rich menu of useful principles, practices, tools and personal competencies, a number of which will be discussed in chapter 6. The following chapter will examine governance in another 'theatre' of public health, that relating to responding to public health emergencies, with a view to assessing the relevance of network governance in that context.

CHAPTER 4

GOVERNANCE IN 'WAR-TIME':
NETWORKS AND PUBLIC HEALTH EMERGENCIES

Introduction

L et us review the path we have followed to this point. The first chapter argued that the public health field is characterized by a high degree of fragmentation, and identified three major fault lines as determinants of this outcome. The second chapter dealt with the notion of network governance and underscored the potential of this model to weave together the efforts of multiple players seeking to achieve common public health objectives.

This chapter will deal with the applicability of the network governance model in the case of public health emergencies and, more specifically, to the response to such events. Intuitively, it can seem fairly self-evident that the response to emergencies requires a strong centralized model of governance. Still, it is worth asking whether network governance is even conceivable in the context of public health emergencies, or whether emergency management by its nature requires resorting to the more traditional hierarchical model of government.

For our discussion of this issue, we will draw from a well-documented and recent event, the SARS crisis of 2003. How were these events perceived from a governance perspective, and what was the prevailing view about how similar events should be dealt with in the future? Tragic as SARS was for a number of individuals in Canada, the crisis and the problematic response to it in Canada, mostly Ontario, served to draw attention to the state of the public health system in Canada, which many felt had been neglected for decades. Three major government reviews were produced to examine these events. One such report, by the National Advisory Committee on SARS and Public Health, commonly referred to as the *Naylor Report*, viewed the events from a national perspective. Two others were commissioned by the Ontario government to look at the issue from the perspective of that province. They were the Expert Panel on SARS and Infectious Disease Control (*Walker Report*) and the SARS Commission (*Campbell Report*). Finally, one report was tabled by the Senate Standing Committee on Social Affairs, Sciences and Technology, which we will refer to as the *Kirby Report*, after its chair, Senator Michael Kirby. In addition to the government and parliamentary reports, papers were written by one of the institutes of the Canadian Institutes of Health Research, by non-governmental organizations, such as the Canadian Medical Association, the Canadian Public Health Association, and by various academics in their own right. Together, this body of literature provides a useful 'window' on the prevailing views about governance in times of public health emergencies.

In many respects, the *ex post facto* analyses of the crisis made useful recommendations which led to a strengthening of public health in Canada. The creation of the Public Health Agency of Canada and the establishment of the Pan-Canadian Public Health Network, discussed in the previous chapter, are examples of these. However, in one respect it injected into the discussion a notion of governance which, if adopted, could prove to be counter-productive to efforts to respond to public health emergencies. Specifically, one observes a somewhat troubling dichotomy in the literature. While a more horizontal style of governance is seen as appropriate and advisable for public health in non-emergency situations, such as health promotion and chronic disease prevention, the governance model prescribed for dealing with emergencies reflects an overall orientation towards a vertically integrated, command-and-control model. We will argue that this dichotomy is in itself problematic, and that applying a command-and-control model to public health emergency situations risks aggravating the problems by adding further layers of complexity to an already complex situation and by damaging relationships that will be necessary for the longer term. As an alternative, we will suggest that a network governance approach, adapted to the particularities of emergency situations, provides what is ultimately a more effective, realistic and sustainable governance model to deal with public health emergency situations. Finally, applying this analysis to the more recent H1N1 pandemic in Canada, we will argue that while valiant efforts were made to use a collaborative approach – notwithstanding the post-SARS reports – a more systematic and rigorous application of a network governance model is needed to respond to pandemic threats in the future.

Brief review of the SARS events

The Severe Acute Respiratory Syndrome (SARS) is a respiratory illness caused by a corona virus. The SARS story has been told many times (see for example Fidler 2004a; *Campbell Report* 2005a), and does not need repeating in detail here. For our purposes, it suffices to recall that the origins of SARS can be located in China in 2002, where there were reports of an outbreak of a mysterious infectious disease. On February 21, 2003, Dr. Liu Jianlun, a physician from Guangdong Province in mainland China travelled to Hong Kong to attend the wedding of a relative. By the time he checked into his hotel, he was feeling unwell. Dr. Liu was admitted to hospital the following day, and died on March 4. An investigation later revealed that during his stay, he infected 12 other guests of the hotel. Among those was a 78 year old woman from Toronto. Shortly after returning to Toronto on February 23, she, too, fell sick and died at home on March 5, with what was diagnosed at the time as a heart attack. Two days later, her son was admitted to the Scarborough Hospital with similar symptoms. Shortly afterward, this individual was placed in isolation, with suspected tuberculosis, but not before coming in contact with several medical staff, other patients and many visitors.

In parallel with the events in Toronto, others who had stayed in the same hotel as the Chinese physician also began feeling unwell. Also, several dozen health care workers at the hospital in Hong Kong where Dr. Liu had been treated were also becoming sick. Beginning to connect the dots that this was a serious outbreak of an infectious disease, the WHO issued a global alert on March 12. Before long, this mysterious and frightening new disease was given a name – Severe Acute Respiratory Syndrome or SARS.

The progression of SARS followed two waves in Toronto. The first is usually set between March 13 and April 23, 2003. During that period, SARS continued to spread at the Scarborough

Hospital. Also during this period, a patient was transferred to York Central Hospital, which started another SARS cluster. More and more people in Toronto were reporting similar symptoms and being admitted to hospital. The three days of March 25-27, combining suspect and probable cases, were the highest three-day period of the outbreak. On March 26, Ontario Premier Ernie Eves declared a provincial emergency and the province activated its Provincial Operations Centre for emergency response. On April 23, the WHO issued a travel advisory against Toronto, Beijing and Shanxi province in China. Ironically, this marks the beginning of the period usually identified as the period between the waves of the disease. From April 24 to May 22, the number of new cases dropped dramatically, and it seemed that the disease had run its course. The WHO lifted the travel advisory on April 30, and on May 14, Toronto was removed from the list of areas with recent local transmission. However, a new wave of reported cases, this time centred at St. John's Rehabilitation Hospital and North York General Hospital, began on May 23 and continued until June 30.

By the time the second outbreak was contained in the fall of 2003, SARS had caused the deaths of 774 people worldwide, of which 44 were located in Canada, all but one in Ontario (Centres for Disease Control and Prevention 2004). While the number of SARS-related deaths was relatively low, the incident highlighted the weak state of Canada's public health infrastructure and led to a broad debate about how the public health in Canada should be strengthened. The general consensus was that this was the "final, tragic wake-up call" (*Campbell Report* 2004: 37) for a public health system that was "broken" in a number of key respects, and if it had not been for the heroic efforts of health professionals, who put at risk their health and that of their families, the number of casualties would have been much higher.

Flawed governance prescriptions in post-SARS literature

The national perspective

The question of intergovernmental roles and responsibilities, as was discussed in chapter 1, is one of the major fault lines characterizing public health governance in Canada. It is natural, therefore for the *Kirby* and *Naylor* reports, which examined the SARS crisis from a national perspective, to focus a considerable amount of attention on the federal/provincial/territorial aspects of the governance issue. In the case of the *Campbell* and *Walker* reports, reviewing the SARS events from the vantage point of a province, specifically Ontario, the concern is primarily with relationships between the provincial level and the local/regional level, although Ontario-federal government relations are also briefly mentioned. Each of these perspectives will be examined in turn.

All four reports agree that the response to SARS was characterized by a significant lack of coordination, resulting from a lack of clarity during the crisis about roles and responsibilities, and which led to confusion, inefficiencies, turf warfare, duplication in some areas and neglect in others (*Kirby Report* 2003: 12). Similarly, there is broad agreement over what should characterize public health governance in cases of infectious disease outbreaks. Although the language used might vary, the writers reflect the need for a response system which is seamless, and in which roles and responsibilities are known in advance and exercised in a coordinated manner.

It is in this context that the intergovernmental relations aspect must be understood. From the national perspective, it is fair to say that Canada's federal system of government is depicted, if not as a 'problem,' at least as a major challenge to overcome. The *Naylor Report* points out that, "[o]ur first theme is that the single largest impediment to dealing successfully with future public health crises is the lack of a collaborative framework and ethos among different levels of government" (*Naylor Report* 2003: 212).

A great deal of attention in the writings is focused on how to overcome the impediments brought by the federal system to deal effectively with public health emergencies. Complicating the picture is the recognition that while the federal government has a role in public health, from its jurisdiction over national emergencies, as well as its spending power and the responsibility for assuring "peace, order, and good government," the actual workings of public health take place largely at the local and provincial levels (Braën 2002).

The starting point for the *Naylor Report*, echoed by the *Kirby Report*, is the importance of building collaboration between federal, provincial and territorial governments as it relates to public health. In fact, one of the major thrusts of the *Naylor Report* is about finding ways to improve federal/provincial/territorial collaboration in the future. The report contains numerous recommendations to establish new ways for federal, provincial and territorial governments to collaborate in all facets of public health, including surveillance, research, chronic disease prevention, and several other areas. In the end, the *Naylor Report* acknowledges that "attempts at unilateral centralization of authority in a fragile federation with a complex division of powers and responsibilities are generally a prescription for conflict, not progress" (*Naylor Report* 2003: 79).

In more 'normal' times, both the *Naylor* and *Kirby* reports propose using incentives, financial and non-financial, to shape the activities at the local and provincial levels and to strengthen existing federal/provincial/territorial mechanisms to achieve a seamless public health system. The *Naylor Report*, for example, recommends the use of "program funding" to provinces and territories "in agreed areas" to strengthen their public health capacity (Ibid.: 215). Similarly, both reports recommend the use of memoranda of understanding, tied to funding, to achieve collaboration within the norms of established federal/provincial/territorial mechanisms (Ibid.: 2003: 164; *Kirby Report* 2003: 45).

On the other hand, the *Naylor* and *Kirby* reports present quite a different governance model for situations of emergency and disaster response. They argue that while collaboration is the goal, it cannot be assumed in emergency situations and that in these cases, a governance model that is reflective of a hierarchical, command-and-control style regime may well be necessary. In order to deal with such circumstances, the two reports recommend the passage of 'default legislation' which, in the event of an emergency, would give the federal government the power to override provincial governments and would impose obligations on provincial and territorial governments as well as municipal governments (*Naylor Report* 2003: 170; *Kirby Report* 2003: 18). While expressing a preference for collaboration and consensus building, the *Naylor Report* points out that these often fail, and that federal health emergency legislation is "a necessary last resort if collaboration and consensus-building mechanisms fail" (*Naylor Report* 2003: 165).

The *Naylor Report* acknowledges existing federal legislation, in the form of the *Emergencies Act*, but states that legislation to deal specifically with public health emergencies would be preferable (Ibid.: 177). This legislation would go so far as to allow the federal government to commandeer provincial and territorial as well as local public health officials "for matters such as disease surveillance," although these powers would be used only when necessary and on a temporary basis (Ibid.: 177).

The literature looking at the SARS crisis from a national perspective, therefore, reveals two governance models. In non-emergency situations, a consensual, collaborative style of governance is seen as the desirable objective. Emergency response, on the other hand, is seen as potentially requiring a much more centralized role played by the federal government in which it assumes a command-and-control role *vis-à-vis* provinces, territories and municipal governments.

The Ontario perspective

A similar dichotomous pattern can be seen in the material dealing with SARS from an Ontario perspective. Although the *Campbell* and *Walker* reports do not focus significantly on the federal government dimension, except to underline the importance of provincial legislation aligning with federal legislation (*Walker Report* 2004: 100), their perception of public health governance seems consistent with those articulated in the *Naylor* and *Kirby* reports. As with the national reports, the two Ontario reports point to poor or non-existent coordination stemming from a lack of a clear definition of respective roles and responsibilities as the key weaknesses to emerge out of the response to SARS. The proposed response to this problem, expressed with particular clarity in the *Campbell Report,* is the need for hierarchical, command-and-control governance in emergency situations. Indeed, both the *Campbell* and the *Walker* reports comment favourably on the consistency of the vision in all four major reports on SARS (*Campbell Report* 2004: 162; *Walker Report* 2004: 69).

The more decentralized, partnership-based approach is not elaborated to any great extent in the SARS-related literature. This is to be expected, since the catalyst for this literature relates to a particular context – an outbreak of a frightening new infectious disease. The *Campbell Report* makes it clear that the mandate of that commission is to focus on SARS and "on infectious diseases as opposed to other public health concerns such as childhood obesity, heart disease, and other aspects of health promotion" (*Campbell Report* 2005a: 82). Nonetheless, this model of governance is referred to in the *Campbell Report,* particularly in the context of health promotion and chronic disease prevention. For example, in the discussion around the question of whether the responsibility, and the funding, for public health should continue to be split between the Ontario government and the municipal governments, or whether it be preferable to upload most or all of the responsibilities to the provincial government, the *Campbell Report* writes:

> *Those medical officers of health who oppose provincial uploading position their argument for local stewardship largely in the nature of health promotion work, which depends on local community partnerships with non-governmental organizations, school boards and other local institutions. The argument is that local stewardship strengthens these partnerships, which would be lost or diminished if the province took over public health* (Ibid.: 88).

The *Campbell Report* goes on to cite a public health official who indicated in an interview:

> *I think public health ...is extremely broad and ...what makes sense perhaps for something like communicable disease control and health protection may have a different balancing in terms of local versus provincial input than is required if you are looking at things that are more community based health promotion* (Ibid.: 89).

In the end, the *Campbell Report* recommends in favour of the uploading option, but makes it very clear that in doing so, it is not dismissing the importance of partnerships at the community level, or of a partnership approach. At one point, this report tries (somewhat unsatisfactorily) to square the circle by stating that "[f]ull tax uploading and full provincial control is perfectly consistent with the continuation of such partnerships" (Ibid.: 94).

The *Walker Report* is somewhat more explicit in articulating the importance of a horizontal, partnership-based model of governance (*Walker Report* 2004: 66, 89). However, its approach to dealing with emergency situations, such as an infectious disease outbreak, is very consistent with what is found in the *Campbell Report*. On this point, both the *Campbell* and the *Walker* reports take a strong position in support of a vertically integrated command-and-control model. Justice Campbell made the case very clearly in writing: "SARS showed us ... that it is essential that one person be in overall charge of our public health defence against infectious outbreaks. While cooperation and teamwork are required in any large endeavour, an effective defence requires that all public health aspects be under the leadership of one person" (*Campbell Report* 2005a: 36-37).

In a similar way to the national reports, which saw the necessity for the federal government to take a strong leadership position with the provinces and territories in periods of crisis, the Ontario studies stress the importance for the province to affirm its leadership position with the municipalities and the regional boards of health. The *Campbell Report* points out that while in "ordinary times" it was acceptable for local medical officers of health to have authority concurrent with the Chief Medical Officer of Health (CMOH) at the provincial level, in health emergencies, one person needs to be clearly in charge (Ibid.: 58). Making the argument that an infectious disease outbreak is no time for turf wars or jurisdictional disputes, Campbell makes a strong case for institutional clarity and simplification to give the CMOH "the authority to direct and ensure an appropriate level of institutional protection against infectious disease" (Ibid.: 183).

Similarly, the *Walker Report* states that: "Ontario needs a single authority on all infection control and communicable disease issues in order to ensure cohesion and continuity throughout the province" (*Walker Report* 2004: 149). The authors writing at the provincial level advocate in favour of stronger legislation to clarify and strengthen the role of the province *vis-à-vis* local/ regional bodies, and making medical officers of health at the local/regional level report directly to the provincial level CMOH (*Campbell Report* 2005a: 18; *Walker Report* 2004: 13).

As with the case of the literature from the national perspective, therefore, what emerges from the Ontario reports is a double-sided view of public health governance. A horizontal, de-centralized model is seen as appropriate in 'ordinary circumstances,' whereas a vertically integrated model is seen as necessary in emergency circumstances.

The intragovernmental dimension

The existence of two models of governance can also be seen in the positioning of public health within the machinery of the government and in the definition of the role of the Chief Public Health Officer (CPHO), federally, or the CMOH, at the provincial level. Taking particular prominence in the four major reports on SARS is a view underlining the importance of providing a certain level of autonomy to the CPHO/CMOH and to the agencies or branches of government that support them. The notion is that public health should be kept at some distance from the regular operations of government (*Kirby Report* 2003: 24; *Naylor Report* 2003: 73; *Walker Report* 2004: 157; *Campbell Rep*ort 2005a: 17; Canadian Institutes of Health Research 2003: 35). The rationale for this is set in the context of what is needed to respond effectively to emergency situations. It follows three interrelated lines of reasoning, which can be described broadly as relating to political, bureaucratic and scientific considerations.

From a political perspective, there is a strong and recurring view of the importance for the CPHO/CMOH to be able to operate free of political interference and, indeed, free of the *perception* of political interference. The concern here is that political leaders may have, or be perceived to have, interests at variance from public health, which could put the public at risk in an emergency. As the *Campbell Report* expressed it: "Any perception that decisions are made for political or economic reasons will sap public confidence and diminish public cooperation. That is why it is so important to have the Chief Medical Officer of Health ...actively and visibly in charge of any public health emergency" (*Campbell Report* 2005a: 252). There is particularly a concern about the area of communications, and the importance for public health leaders to be able to communicate freely with the public in an emergency, unconstrained by extraneous considerations (*Naylor Report* 2003: 76-7; *Campbell Report* 2005a: 339).

Second, there is a view that regular government bureaucracies are process-oriented and therefore too slow and cumbersome to respond effectively in emergency situations. There is also a perceived risk that regular government bureaucracies are more likely to be influenced by political considerations (*Naylor Report* 2003: 72; *Walker Report* 2004: 78).

Finally, the argument is made that having the public health agency or branch working at some distance from the regular governmental bureaucracy would help to ensure that decisions within the agency in question are made on the basis of science, and not for reasons unrelated to public health. The reasoning appears to be that public health professionals, working at arm's length from the regular bureaucracy, would be able to avoid the murky world of policy and politics and instead base their conclusions and their actions on good science (*Naylor Report* 2003: 73). Perhaps the most succinct articulation of this perspective can be found in the Canadian Medical Association's submission to the Senate Standing Committee on Social Affairs, Science and Technology, which stated bluntly: "Science and health protection must trump politics" (Canadian Medical Association 2003a).

The literature examining public health from a national perspective is not completely unanimous on the means to achieve greater autonomy for the public health function, with the *Naylor* and the *Kirby* reports recommending a separate federal department led by a chief public health officer and the CMA opting for a federal arm's length agency (*Kirby Report* 2003: 32-3). There is, nonetheless, a high level of consistency on the objectives to be attained. At the provincial level, the *Walker Report* took a more nuanced approach, putting forward options which balanced the autonomy of the CMOH with the level of autonomy of the public health agency, so that if the CMOH had formal legal authority to speak on urgent public health matters, then the need for autonomy of the public health branch from the ministry was diminished (*Walker Report* 2004: 91). Here again, however, there is no disagreement between the *Walker* and the *Campbell* reports on the end result of a public health function operating autonomously or semi-autonomously from the regular structures and operations of government.

This depiction of intragovernmental relations in the four reports, as it relates to the response to health emergencies, is quite consistent with a vertically integrated model of governance. It is designed to ensure speed in decision making by one, or at least a very small number of actors, with public health expertise. Unlike in the world of modern governance, there is no question here about who is in charge.

Concurrent with this view, there also is a concern that public health structures avoid becoming isolated within government. Several of the reports following SARS point to the need for intersectoral relationships within government to arrive at public policies which are conducive to public health, but may be found outside the health sector. Speaking of the role of the CMOH, the *Campbell Report* stated that he/she should be at the table within government, rather than being "a watchdog off in a corner" (*Campbell Report* 2005a: 20). The *Kirby Report* makes a similar point in saying "...it is clear that the health of Canadians cannot be protected by the health system working in isolation.

The action or inaction of many other sectors greatly influences our health" (*Kirby Report* 2003: 32). The *Naylor Report* also refers to "the need to ensure integration of public health activity with a wide variety of departments, not least, Health Canada itself" (*Naylor Report* 2003: 74).

Although the authors do not explore the issue beyond recognizing the importance of maintaining the horizontal capacity, the skills and the organizational design related to this activity are quite different from those consistent with a more vertical organization. Horizontal management requires building relationships with other governmental entities, rather than constructing a semi-autonomous edifice. Far from wanting to remove public health from the regular workings of government, the objective here is to make public health more of a player in government decision making (*Campbell Report* 2005a: 344). Furthermore, rather than concentrating on the relationships between health professionals, horizontal management requires building linkages with other policy sectors, which have interests and objectives of their own, but which can be allied to health policy objectives.

As with intergovernmental relationships, therefore, the view of intragovernmental relationships in the four major reports implicitly suggests the coexistence of two different models of governance. How can these be reconciled? The vertically integrated model appears to coincide quite clearly with the view of the authors about what is needed in times of public health emergencies. Although this is not elaborated to any great extent, one infers the view that in between emergencies, the public health apparatus needs to operate in a broader, more inclusive manner. The distinction seems to be between how public health emergencies behave in 'peace-time,' as opposed to when they are responding in times of crisis, such as posed by a pandemic.

Outside of the government and parliamentary reports, a similar pattern can also be seen in the writings of others in the public health community about the SARS response and the measures needed to prepare for future public health emergencies. Kumanan Wilson and Harvey Lazar, for example, recognize that local public health officials constitute the "backbone" of public health and acknowledge that it is, therefore, important, in developing public health strategies, to avoid alienating provincial and local public health officials (Wilson and Lazar 2005: 17). Yet the authors argue strongly that the federal government cannot rely on the collaborative approach with provinces and territories, and advocate "a re-definition of federal capacity to respond to public health emergencies" (Ibid.: 6). Among other powers, the authors argue that the federal government "needs the ability to acquire complete knowledge of an outbreak," on the grounds that an infectious disease cannot be managed without comprehensive surveillance data, and that it should therefore have the authority to bypass provincial governments and deal directly with local governments" (Ibid.: 14).[12] Similar to the *Naylor Report*, this capacity would include the power to override provincial governments and if necessary commandeer provincial and local staff (Ibid.: 19; Wilson 2006: 38). At the very least, the authors see the existence of heavy weaponry in the federal arsenal as having the effect of inciting provincial and territorial governments to collaborate, which could be seen as an attempt to bridge the two models of governance (Wilson and Lazar 2005: 21).

Similar to what is advocated in relation to intergovernmental relationships, the apparent dichotomy of governance models appears to be based on an assumption that while public health needs to be broad-based and inclusive, emergency situations require a command-and-control response to avoid confusion about roles and to allow for clear decision making. But is the latter part of the assumption necessarily accurate? As the next section will discuss, the assumption that command-and-control models are necessary in emergencies, and that such crises necessarily preclude applications of network governance can and should be questioned.

Can network governance be applied to emergencies?

The response to the SARS events should not be surprising. Emergency situations, and fears of emergencies, typically generate a strong desire for hierarchy and centralization (Waugh

[12] One of the frequently cited rationales for a centralized approach in Canada derives from the global context of public health and disease outbreaks. As Wilson and Lazar put it: "Canada's roles and responsibilities as part of the larger international community provide compelling reasons for a re-evaluation of the current federal approach to public health emergencies" (Wilson and Lazar 2005: 13). As the national government, Canada would be expected to report to the WHO the information needed for the global management of an infectious disease outbreak. Failure to do so could have serious consequences, such as the imposition of a WHO travel advisory.

and Streib 2006: 138). The public wants to be reassured that someone is 'in charge' of the situation. This same response can be witnessed around the response to the H1N1 pandemic of 2009. In an editorial in the *Canadian Medical Association Journal* (CMAJ), Paul Hebert and Noni Macdonald indicated that the Public Health Agency of Canada, as presently constituted, and the position of the Chief Public Health Officer, are insufficient, and that what is needed is an independent health "czar," "with executive powers across all jurisdictions and who is ultimately accountable to the highest office in the country" (*Canadian Medical Association Journal* 2009). In a similar vein, Professor Peter McKenna recently argued that: "It goes without saying that there should not be different inoculation programs right across the country. This is one of those rare occasions in a federation where the central government needs to step to the front of the line and override provincial autonomy" (McKenna 2009).

Notwithstanding these reactions, the calls for greater centralization fail to take into consideration the real achievements of collaborative practices in emergencies and, if acted upon, threaten to compound the problem, rather than addressing it (Waugh and Streib 2006: 138). There is increasing evidence, based on case studies, that suggests that the model of centralized hierarchical authority proves in the end to be ineffective and counterproductive. With specific reference to the Canadian public health context, this can be argued from a number of levels, as follows.

Attempts to simplify may complicate

Paradoxically, attempts at what is often called "institutional simplification" may mean adding yet another level to what already exists, thus further complicating the environment. A new set of rules and structures adds more infrastructure to what is already in place, thus adding to the confusion and ultimately making it more difficult to decide on a course of action and act on it (Koppenjan and Klijn 2004: 9). As Boin and 't Hart have observed: "At the political strategic level, efforts to radically centralize decision-making authority tend to cause more friction than they resolve because they disturb well-established authority patterns" (Boin and 't Hart 2003: 547). In Canada, efforts by the federal government to attempt to unilaterally direct provincial/ territorial and local governments would clearly "disturb well-established authority patterns," and would almost certainly lead to friction and resistance. The notion expressed in the *Naylor Report* and by Wilson and Lazar that the mere threat of unilateral federal action powered by new legislative powers would act as an incentive for provincial and territorial governments to collaborate is, at a minimum, untested and highly risky. A far more likely scenario would be constitutional challenges through the courts by at least some of the provinces, and increased federal/provincial/territorial tensions. The final result could well confirm Koppenjan and Klijn's proposition that attempts at top-down steering create more problems than they resolve.

The threat of collateral damage

Tampering with institutional design can also damage trust relations between the parties, which can have long-term consequences (Koppenjan and Klijn 2004: 232). One could expect that the imposition of centralized authority could damage broader federal, provincial and territorial relations in Canada, which are often fragile, even in more stable periods. Although a public health crisis, such as an outbreak of an infectious disease, would be a matter of serious concern to everyone, it is easily imaginable that policy communities outside the health sector would have legitimate interests that may differ from and perhaps compete with health issues (Boin and 't Hart 2003: 546). Given sensitivities in Canada over matters of jurisdiction, it is likely that provinces and territories, as well as local governments and others, would not welcome the prospect of the Government of Canada determining their priorities, even in the short-term. Resentment from such actions could affect relationships in other (non-health) aspects of federal/provincial/territorial relations, particularly if the issue is carried into the discussion at the more strategic level of federal/provincial/territorial relationships (see chapter 1). As Koppenjan and Klijn have observed succinctly: "The bill for strategic misbehaviour in one game will become due in another." (Koppenjan and Klijn 2004: 57).

How to enforce?

Another point that is raised in the literature refers to the availability, or lack of such, of mechanisms to enforce the imposition of a top-down authority structure in a network environment. In other words, what would be the practicalities of implementing a public health command-and-control operation to manage a public health emergency in Canada? The public health community in Canada is a very diverse community composed of governments at various levels, health professionals, such as physicians, nurses, researchers, non-governmental and voluntary sector organizations, hospitals, clinics, laboratories and several other stakeholders "whose legitimacy is derived from alternative authority sources" as Drabek and McEntire (2003) have put it. It hardly seems realistic to attempt to impose a rigid command-and-control structure on this community over a sustained period. Boin and 't Hart, for example, speculate that actors "whose policy-making roles are abruptly diminished by the *ad hoc* centralization of authority will, to say the least, not be motivated to contribute their resources and comply with centrally issued policy directives" (Boin and 't Hart 2003: 547). How would the directives of such a structure be enforced and what sanctions or penalties could be imposed on jurisdictions who refused to "fall in line"? Finally, from a practical perspective, one wonders how realistic it is that the federal government would be able to commandeer provincial staff, as Wilson and Lazar proposed (Wilson and Lazar 2005: 19). How would the federal government ensure compliance from provincial/territorial staff? Would the federal government even have the capacity to manage such an enterprise, particularly if it had to be implemented on short notice? A serious consideration of these questions leads to doubt that attempting to centralize management of an infectious disease crisis in Canada is, in any way, realistic.

Pre-crisis preparation requires trust

The literature on emergency planning and response identifies four essential elements in the process: hazard mitigation; preparedness; response; and recovery. (Waugh and Streib 2006: 131; Drabek and McEntire 2003: 98; Petak 1985: 3). Hazard mitigation refers to all measures that can be taken to prevent or lessen the impact of an occurrence. Preparedness includes the planning activities, to ensure that people are trained on what to do in a crisis and that systems and resources (human, financial and physical) are in place when they are needed. The point is regularly made that pre-crisis activities are key to managing an emergency successfully (Waugh and Streib 2006: 132; Tam et al. 2005: 406). Furthermore, it is essential that these preparations involve all those who would have a part in dealing with such an occurrence, since a large part of the preparedness phase involves the coordination of a wide range of actors and resources (Boin and 't Hart 2003: 547). To succeed, this work needs to be inclusive and collaborative.

It is highly doubtful that a radical shift could be made from an inclusive, collaborative pre-crisis stage to a hierarchical command-and-control model in a crisis. In the Canadian public health context, the federal government would need a hidden "plan B" to be used in the event of a crisis, the very existence of which could probably not be kept secret for long, and which could damage collaborative efforts to prepare for a crisis. Indeed, trust, which is consistently highlighted in the literature as one of the essential ingredients for successful collaboration (see chapter 9), would almost certainly be an early casualty. Far from the threat of federal unilateral action being an incentive for provinces and territories, and possibly others, to take direction from the federal government, that threat, whether tacit or explicit, might well provoke those jurisdictions to do just the opposite.

The need for flexibility and inclusiveness

The four elements of emergency preparedness and response require the involvement of a large number of actors, many of whom, as stated above, derive their authority from different sources (Waugh and Streib 2006: 134; Boin and 't Hart 2003: 547). Furthermore, crises are often very fluid events, with rapidly changing circumstances. In these circumstances, "pivotal policy decisions actually emerge from a multi-actor coordination process, in which consultation, negotiation, and outright confrontation are the orders of the day" (Boin and 't Hart 2003: 547; see also Moynihan 2009; Drabek and McEntire 2003: 107). Even in a crisis, leadership terms must often be negotiated (Moynihan 2009: 2; Waugh and Streib 2006: 133). What is required in an emergency is flexibility and agility. Yet the command-and-control model tends to be overly rigid, precisely the opposite of what is needed in this context (Drabek and McEntire 2003: 107).

Harnessing the potential of existing networks

Waugh and Streib have made the point that it is a mistake to assume that any individual or organization can manage all the relief and recovery efforts during a catastrophic disaster (Waugh and Streib 2006: 134). Capacity is clearly one part of this. It is highly questionable whether the federal government would have the capacity necessary to manage provincial/territorial and local staff that would be commandeered to deal with a public health emergency. But perhaps more fundamental is the issue of having the necessary knowledge to manage all aspects of a crisis. Moynihan points out that for most emergencies: "(t)he response is likely to demand such a wide variety of expertise, knowledge, and number of respondents that no single public agency has the resources to comprehensively tackle the emergency" (Moynihan 2005: 8).

In Canada, the knowledge required would mean, not only having the full scientific picture, but also knowing the particular players and particular circumstances in each region of Canada. Given the significantly regionalized nature of Canada, and the fact that public health is primarily a matter that falls under provincial jurisdiction, a very high level of interregional variation is to be expected. It is highly questionable that a single actor or organization would to be able to capture this knowledge and apply it effectively. On the other hand, it is critically important that managers recognize that they are operating in a network environment, and know how to capitalize on the resources those networks can provide to help deal with a crisis. As Waugh and Streib point out, "improved performance in emergency management depends to a great extent on the ability of public officials to fully comprehend the complexities of the policy networks operating in the areas in which they work and to think strategically about how to use them" (Waugh and Streib 2006: 138).

Science does NOT trump politics

Contrary to the CMA position that "science and health protection must trump politics," the reality is that there are a number of other crucial factors that are involved besides pure science. Psychology, organizational behaviour, regional cultures and political science also play major roles as do the public policy decision-making processes, which legitimately includes elected officials. Because of its need to interact with the population, and because of its link to government, public health "is inherently political by nature" (Corber 2007: 42).[13]

---

[13] In sharp contrast with the view that scientific evidence alone should determine public policy, the American political scientist, Aaron Wildavsky, stated: ... political rationality is the fundamental kind of reason because it deals with the preservation and improvement of decision structures, and decision structures

It is of course important to ensure that proposed courses of action are supported, where possible, by sound evidence and that science be used to avoid what some observers have called "negotiated nonsense." At the same time, it is essential to appreciate the complexity of today's decision-making environment and to recognize that science, on its own, can influence but not predetermine policy outcomes.

What style of leadership?

A related point is the type of leadership that is needed in an emergency. Contrary to the "commander in chief" model advocated in the post-SARS literature, the literature on emergency response suggests that what is needed is a more flexible leadership style that is adaptive and that encourages the sharing of information, organizational learning and collaboration. Waugh and Streib point out that:

> The leadership strategy required for crises may well be counterintuitive. Information often flows from the bottom in a traditional hierarchy, to the extent that it flows at all. Such a situation may be better handled by a style that is affiliative, open, and democratic. An authoritarian response would certainly be faster and more consistent, but it would require insight and vision that may not be available to those with actual authority and media access (Waugh and Streib 2006: 136).

Without question, leadership is a key element in responding to a crisis. Critical factors, however, are the style of leadership that is used, as well as the positioning of this leadership. With regard to the former, it is important to recognize that in an emergency, it is not possible for one person to "fully command attention or to compel compliance" (Ibid.: 138). Rather than an authoritarian leadership model, what is more effective is leadership based on strategic thinking and the ability to communicate and negotiate with others (Huxham and Vangen 2000; Waugh and Streib 2006; Moynihan 2009).

Where the leadership is located is also important. Unlike in the more hierarchical and bureaucratic models, the emergency

---

are the sources of all decisions...There can be no conflict between political rationality and...technical, legal, social, or economic rationality, because the solution of political problems makes possible an attack on any other problems, while a serious political deficiency can prevent or undo all other problem solving (cited in Rhodes and Wanna, 2007: 419).

manager does not have to be the most senior member of the largest organization. In fact, in some organizations, the manager is not even an employee of the 'senior' organization. At times, this person is chosen by representatives of all the jurisdictions involved. As will be discussed below in the context of the incident command system (ICS), even when a manager/commander has been selected, member organizations retain a certain amount of their autonomy, meaning that the leader is less than a 'commander' in the traditional sense, and more of a coordinator/ facilitator (Moynihan 2009: 13).

Taking stock

With respect to emergency preparedness and response, Drabek and McEntire conclude that: "The command and control model is ...based on inadequate theory, incomplete evidence and a weak methodology" (Drabek and McEntire 2003: 106). If the traditional/ hierarchical model is not appropriate for dealing with emergency situations, how realistic is it to think that a network governance model would work better? This question has been the subject of debate for some time. For the past several decades, there has been an increasing level of support for a model that favours cooperation and communication. The command-and-control model tends to surface periodically in reaction to an event that has taken place, such as the events around September 11, 2001 and Hurricane Katrina in the US, where some seek the assurance of having someone 'in charge' in the event of a crisis (Waugh and Streib 2006: 132). The same phenomenon has been witnessed in Canada around the SARS crisis and to a lesser extent, the H1N1 pandemic. Yet, as Waugh and Streib have argued, this sort of thinking "is inconsistent with the tenets of the field and displays blindness to what collaborative action has accomplished" (Ibid.: 138) The network governance model, on the other hand, provides a more promising avenue to combine the benefits of a collaborative model with the exigencies of emergency situations (Moynihan 2009: 17). While it rests on the foundation of collaborative principles, it also attempts to build a structure around how autonomous organizations interrelate in dealing with a crisis.

Network governance in the context of emergency response has been operationalized by the incident command system (ICS). First conceived in the United States in 1970s for the purpose of fighting forest fires in California, the "goal of the ICS is to provide a hierarchical framework upon which to manage the network of agencies involved" (Moynihan 2009: 32). ICS might look on the surface like a traditional command-and-control model, yet "it is better understood as a highly centralized mode of network governance, designed to coordinate interdependent responders under urgent conditions" (Ibid.: 2). While it recognizes the need for an onsite commander or manager, it does not require the participating organizations to cede any jurisdictional control. Moreover, while the title seems to imply otherwise, the role of 'commander' incorporates the need for collaborating with other members and negotiating policy decisions wherever possible rather than imposing them. Under the ICS, "the legitimacy of command is negotiated among network members" (Ibid.: 2).

In the United States, the Federal Emergency Management Agency (FEMA) went from a hierarchical organization to a network model in the mid-1990s. As Kettl points out: "FEMA ...moved from a limited form of direct service delivery to a complex, network-based approach that stretched from the federal government into state and local governments and the private sector" (Kettl 2000: 495) Similarly, the Department of Homeland Security uses ICS for all crisis situations (Moynihan 2009: 1). Moreover, both the National Incident Management System (NIMS) and the National Response Plan use ICS as a central feature (Ibid.: 3). The NIMS explicitly recognizes that for most major emergencies, a network will be required (Ibid.: 8). As part of this approach, the American federal government role has been changed, "from being the proverbial cavalry, rushing in to save people, to being a supporter of individual and community efforts to reduce risks and prepare for and respond to disasters" (Waugh and Streib 2006: 135). An interview with a senior official from Public Safety Canada, which has the mandate to deal with national emergencies, confirmed that in Canada, a similar approach has been adopted by that department (Interview #52: February 8, 2010).

Although the ICS, as a form of implementing network governance in emergency situations may sound idealistic, it has been applied and generally found to be successful, with the possible exception of the response to Hurricane Katrina. Waugh and Streib state that: "What we now call the *new governance process* forms the core of our national emergency response. Consensual processes are the rule" (Waugh and Streib 2006: 133). There exists broad consensus that agencies with different areas of specialty and accountabilities need to find a way to organize and cooperate, and that the ICS provides a useful mechanism for accomplishing that objective. At the same time, it must be recognized that the ICS does not provide an exact formula that can be applied uniformly in all circumstances. Indeed, a large part of its success will be to adapt to the organizational cultures of those participating in each case. For example, as Waugh and Streib point out, public health professionals, "generally expect open discussion of issues before decisions" (Ibid.: 134). This leads to the question of how network governance generally and, ICS in particular, can be applied to the particular circumstances of public health.

Although there are several case studies on the use of ICS in emergency situations, there are few of which we are aware that deal with situations involving public health. Perhaps the closest approximation is the case which Donald P. Moynihan has documented about the outbreak of Exotic Newcastle Disease (END) in 2002-03 (Moynihan 2005). END is an infectious disease which affects poultry and other birds but which is not harmful to humans. It was first detected in California, but spread to 5 different states before it was controlled. It involved 10 major state and federal agencies. In all, 7,000 workers worked on the task force created to stop the spread of the disease.

According to Moynihan, it was clear from the beginning that no single organization had the resources to cope with this outbreak on its own, and therefore working as a network was a necessity. Fortunately, a 'latent' network was already in existence and operated primarily in a 'pre-planning' capacity. Once it was recognized that the disease had broken out, the parties involved decided quickly to become an active network, and adopted the ICS model. A hierarchy was established within the network to allow for faster decision making. Managers were designated with a clear mandate to coordinate and direct the work that needed to be done. In this way, the managers were given a stronger measure of authority than might be seen in networks during non-emergency periods. Even here, however, Moynihan remarks that the managers had to perform their role with a degree of moderation, knowing that the workers involved were ultimately accountable to their home organizations, not the task force. In the end, although problems arose along the way that had to be dealt with, the ICS model was generally seen to be successful (Moynihan 2005: 26).

Emergency preparedness and response in the Canadian context

In Canada, the network model is the model in use at the national level to deal with health emergency preparedness and response (Interview #44: July 7, 2010; Interview #51: December 8, 2009; Interview #35: October 26, 2010). Interestingly, despite the recommendations of the reports discussed earlier, the SARS events have not led, at the national level at least, to a greater centralization of powers and resources. One key informant said simply, "command-and-control would not work in Canada" (Interview #55: July 14, 2011). On the contrary, what Canada has witnessed is the further development of intergovernmental networks to deal with emergencies (Interview #25: March 3, 2011). Early attempts were made in the late 1990s and the early years of the 2000s to draft a proposed federal/provincial/territorial agreement called the National Health Emergency Management System, based on the ICS model. Among other elements, it detailed how the incident commander was to be selected, and described where a single command was to be used, and where a unified command, involving a number of parties, was more appropriate. This document underwent a number of revisions, including a change in title to the Pan-Canadian Health Emergency Management System, and was formally approved by health ministers in 2004 (Interview #51: December 8, 2009). Notwithstanding this, some jurisdictions continued to be uncomfortable with the centralizing language, and with any notion of command-and-control by the federal government (Interview #35: October 26, 2010).

What has emerged as a replacement to a formalized national agreement is more broadly a common understanding among federal, provincial and territorial public health authorities to work together in the event of a health emergency that goes beyond the borders of a single province. Based on this, a number of protocols or memoranda of understanding (MOU) have been and are being negotiated to deal with health emergencies, increasingly taking an all-hazards approach. There are, for example, MOUs on information-sharing and on mutual aid in the event of an emergency, which have been developed and approved by all jurisdictions (Interview #35: October 26, 2010). Because they avoid using the broad language on incident command-and-control, these agreements are proving to be more acceptable to the parties involved. In the end, what has emerged is a network model in which federal, provincial and territorial governments work together to address a health emergency which affects them all, and in a fashion which respects their jurisdictional authority to make decisions they consider appropriate for their circumstances.

Consistent with a network approach, the role of the federal government, particularly the Public Health Agency of Canada, consists largely of coordination and facilitation. The Emergency Manager for the H1N1 pandemic took the role of a 'symphony conductor' of an orchestra playing from a common score sheet. As part of this, PHAC takes a leadership role in developing national guidelines, in close consultation with the other jurisdictions, although provinces and territories can choose whether or not they wish to apply them. PHAC will also seek to enable inter-jurisdictional mutual aid, involving human resources, supplies, and equipment. More broadly, PHAC enables interjurisdictional – interprovincially and across the Canada-US border – transfer of aid needed during an emergency. Training is also made available by PHAC. In addition, through the National Emergency Stockpile System (NESS), the federal agency provides emergency supplies and equipment at the request of the province or territory (Interview #35: October 26, 2010).

Regional cross-border public health collaboration functions between provinces and neighbouring states of the US, covering the eastern states, Great Lakes, and Pacific North-West regions. These have used the templates provided by the International Health Regulations to develop approaches for mutual aid and risk assessment. Furthermore, these three collaborations, as well as three non-aligned provinces and states (Manitoba, Alberta and North Dakota) along with the Canadian and American federal governments, participate in the Canada-US Pan-Border Public Health Preparedness Council which seeks to strengthen capacity on both sides of the border to deal with public health threats and to provide support and enhance coordination between the various regional collaborations (Interview #55: July 14, 2011; http://www.pbphpc.org).

The deepening extent of the networked emergency preparedness and response sector can also be seen by the involvement of voluntary sector organizations (VSOs). The

Council of Emergency Voluntary Sector Services Directors includes such prominent members as the Canadian Red Cross, St. John's Ambulance and the Salvation Army. Also involved is the Council of Emergency Social Services Directors. These organizations are involved in emergency preparedness at every level, with particular emphasis at the local level (Interview #55: July 14, 2011). PHAC recognizes the importance of these organizations by providing the secretariat for this council, as well as providing resources for their face-to face meetings (Interview #35: October 26, 2010; Interview #49: July 7, 2010).

With regard to health emergencies due specifically to pandemics, the Canadian Pandemic Influenza Plan for the Health Sector was negotiated in 2004, in the aftermath of SARS, and updated in 2006. This plan provides a broad framework for a collaborative response to a pandemic. It involves, beyond federal/provincial/territorial governments, chief medical officers of health, public health professionals, such as epidemiologists, virologists, and laboratory specialists; and a large group of stakeholders, such as VSOs, local governments, emergency planners and bioethicists. In addition to this, in 2007 the Public Health Network (see chapter 3) established the Pandemic Influenza Committee, and later the Pandemic Coordination Committee, to provide a central coordinating body for pandemic influenza (Interview #25: March 3, 2011).

The H1N1 pandemic in Canada: What did this reveal?

From the above, it is apparent that Canada had quite extensive infrastructure in place to respond to a pandemic. However, when the H1N1 pandemic struck, it was decided to put in place a new time-limited emergency management structure led by federal/provincial/territorial deputy ministers of health (CDMH) (Public Health Agency of Canada 2010: 35). This committee took responsibility for core functions such as planning, operations, logistics, communications and health services, with individual DMs being assigned to different areas, and assuming the responsibility to report back to their counterparts on emerging issues in that area. A number of federal/provincial/territorial groups were then formed to support the CDMH. Particularly central was the Special Advisory Committee on H1N1, which was composed of members of the PHN Council as well as the

Council of Chief Medical Officers of Health.[14] The role of this committee was to provide strategic policy advice to the CDMH (Ibid.: 36). Next, a number of groups were assigned to support the Special Advisory Committee, in particular, the Pandemic Coordination Committee which had responsibility for the more operational aspects of the response and which was heavily involved in preparing for the second wave. This, in turn, was supported by time-limited task groups, covering such areas as surveillance, epidemiology and laboratories; pandemic vaccines, public health measures; remote and isolated communities; zoonoses, infection control and clinical care and antivirals. Finally, the pre-existing PHN expert and issue groups (see chapter 3) were at various times involved in supporting the Pandemic Coordination Committee, in particular the Canadian Public Health Laboratories Network, the Communicable Disease Control Expert Group, the Surveillance and Information Expert Group, and the Emergency Preparedness and Response Expert Group (Ibid.: 37) Some confusion arose, however, as members of pre-existing groups at times felt side-lined by the new structures and became unsure of their roles (Interview #55: July 14, 2011). A chart illustrating the federal, provincial and territorial emergency management structures for the H1N1 pandemic is shown as Figure 3.

---

[14] There is a significant level of overlap between these two committees (see chapter 3).

FIGURE 3: Emergency Management Structure for H1N1 Pandemic

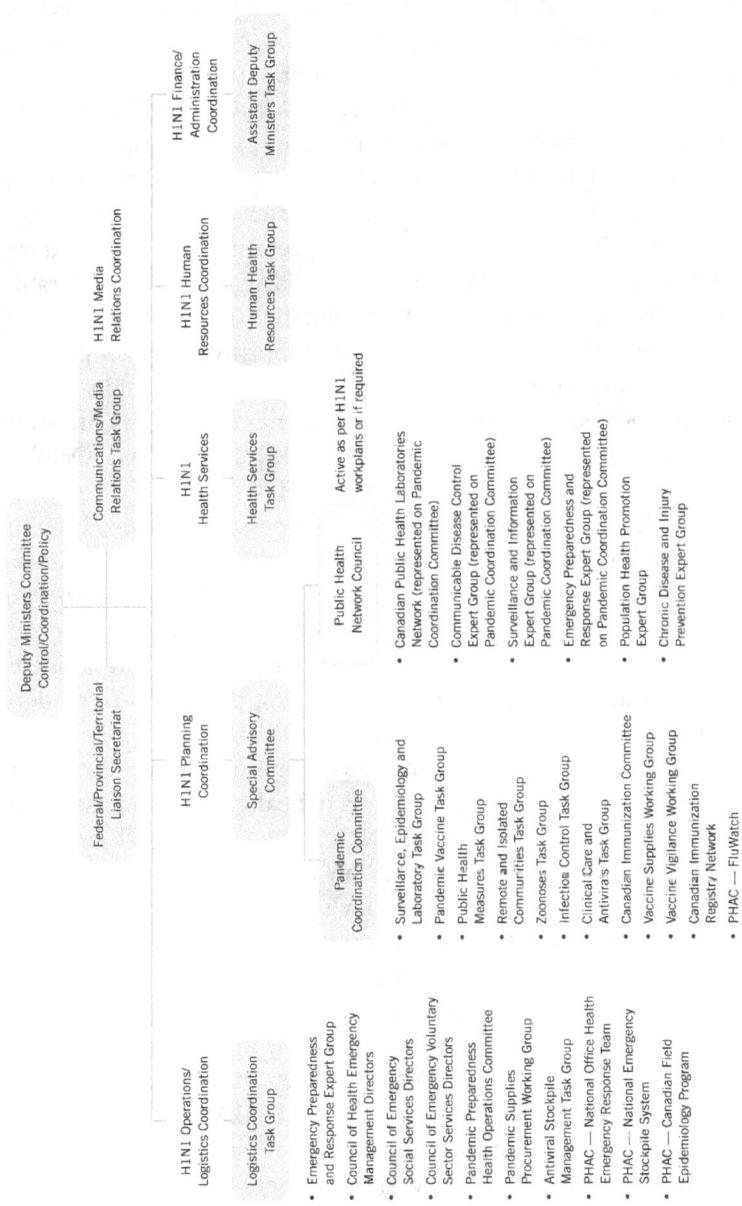

Deputy Ministers Committee Control/Coordination/Policy

H1N1 Finance/Administration Coordination
— Assistant Deputy Ministers Task Group

Communications/Media Relations Task Group

H1N1 Media Relations Coordination

H1N1 Human Resources Coordination
— Human Health Resources Task Group

H1N1 Health Services
— Health Services Task Group (Active as per H1N1 workplans or if required)

Federal/Provincial/Territorial Liaison Secretariat

H1N1 Planning Coordination

Special Advisory Committee

Public Health Network Council
- Canadian Public Health Laboratories Network (represented on Pandemic Coordination Committee)
- Communicable Disease Control
- Communicable Disease Control Expert Group (represented on Pandemic Coordination Committee)
- Surveillance and Information Expert Group (represented on Pandemic Coordination Committee)
- Emergency Preparedness and Response Expert Group (represented on Pandemic Coordination Committee)
- Population Health Promotion Expert Group
- Chronic Disease and Injury Prevention Expert Group

Pandemic Coordination Committee
- Surveillance, Epidemiology and Laboratory Task Group
- Pandemic Vaccine Task Group
- Public Health Measures Task Group
- Remote and Isolated Communities Task Group
- Zoonoses Task Group
- Infection Control Task Group
- Clinical Care and Antivirals Task Group
- Canadian Immunization Committee
- Vaccine Supplies Working Group
- Vaccine Vigilance Working Group
- Canadian Immunization Registry Network
- PHAC — FluWatch

H1N1 Operations/Logistics Coordination

Logistics Coordination Task Group
- Emergency Preparedness and Response Expert Group
- Council of Health Emergency Management Directors
- Council of Emergency Social Services Directors
- Council of Emergency Voluntary Sector Services Directors
- Pandemic Preparedness Health Operations Committee
- Pandemic Supplies Procurement Working Group
- Antiviral Stockpile Management Task Group
- PHAC — National Office Health Emergency Response Team
- PHAC — National Emergency Stockpile System
- PHAC — Canadian Field Epidemiology Program

Source: Lessons Learned Review: Public Health Agency of Canada Response to the 2009 H1N1 Pandemic. *Ottawa: Public Health Agency of Canada and Health Canada, 2010, page 38. Reproduced with permission of the Minister of Health, 2012.*

The H1N1 case is instructive from a number of perspectives. First, it demonstrates a strong commitment to collaboration, particularly from the federal/provincial/ territorial perspective. One informant, who had played a key part in the response, characterized the level of federal/provincial/territorial coordination as "immense" (Interview #35: October 26, 2010). All the major products developed in the course of the pandemic, such as the national guidelines on various aspects of the pandemic response, were put through only after extensive consultations with provincial and territorial representatives. The federal government, particularly through PHAC, took a leadership role, consisting primarily of coordination and facilitation. Key informants interviewed reported an impressive unity of purpose in the response, which allowed participants to put aside, at least for the period of the crisis, jurisdictional differences, in order to deal with the critical issues at hand (Interview #35: October 26, 2010; Interview #25: March 3, 2011).

At the same time, significant weaknesses were also brought to light. To begin with, as was mentioned in chapter 2, networks operate "in the show of hierarchy." Indeed, reconciling the flexibility required in network governance with the strictures of government bureaucracy as it is currently established is one of the central challenges of operationalizing the notion of modern governance. This tension is clearly in evidence in the response to H1N1. One can legitimately question, for example, whether it was necessary for the deputy ministers of health to put themselves in control of the response, when the infrastructure which had been established to prepare for such an event, and which had been agreed to by all parties, did not include this mechanism.

Second, key informants complained that the long chain of approvals required for briefing materials and decision making in 'peace-time' was maintained, leading to numerous delays at critical times, and creating a significant level of frustration for those involved (Interview #28: February 18, 2011; Interview #35: October 26, 2010; Interview #55: July 14, 2011). For example, the situation reports produced by the Emergency Manager, which are only useful for a very short period before they become overtaken by events, required the approval of the ADM, and were particularly scrutinized when they touched on federal/ provincial/territorial relations. This often meant that these reports were of little value by the time they were released (Interview #55: July 14, 2011). The point here is that while command-and-control was not part of the federal/provincial/territorial mechanism at play, it was maintained within the federal health bureaucracy (and possibly within some provincial/territorial health bureaucracies), which did not serve the parties well during the crisis.

A possible indicator of the hierarchical nature of the response to the pandemic within the federal bureaucracy is the number of briefings that were held within the federal health bureaucracy, and the federal bureaucracy in general. The *Lessons Learned Review* points to the fact that over a period of 171 calendar days during the pandemic response, eight PHAC senior managers attended a total of 1,030 meetings and briefings, most of which were internal to the federal government. These included: health portfolio Executive Group meetings (141); briefings with the Minister of Health (94); and 71 meetings of the "Four Corners" group, which included the Minister of Health's office; the Privy Council Office; the Prime Minister's Office; Public Safety Canada; and the Minister of Public Safety's office (Public Health Agency of Canada 2010: 80). On top of this, senior managers were still required to attend regular meetings on subjects not related to the pandemic. The situation facing senior managers in Health Canada was much the same. Again, questions arise about whether this need to satisfy the demands of the internal governmental machinery is consistent with the need to act quickly and flexibly in the event of a crisis.

Partially related to the above point, there seemed to be insufficient attention paid to what some have called 'metagovernance' in network situations – in other words, how to 'manage' the networks that have been put in place, as well as one's own participation in those groups.[15] In the course of the pandemic, it was discovered that there were cases of duplication and confusion between the roles and mandates of some of the new committees and working groups, and those of pre-existing committees (Ibid.: 40) To attempt to correct this, some refinements to the governance structure were made in the interval between the first and second waves (Interview #25: March 3, 2011). Still, the *Lessons Learned Review* documents that a number of provincial and territorial partners, as well as professional associations such

---

[15] Metagovernance will be discussed in chapter 8.

as the Canadian Medical Association and the College of Family Physicians of Canada, questioned the need for the number of working groups and committees that were established, and expressed concern about duplication (Ibid.: 39). This may well have led federal/provincial/territorial deputy ministers of health to agree, at their January 2010 meeting, that "improvements to the governance structure should be continued, with the understanding that any structures would need to be flexible enough to adapt to different types of emergent situations that could affect the health sector and be in place immediately, while respecting jurisdictional responsibilities and authorities" (Ibid.: 39).

Finally, while intense efforts were made to develop intergovernmental networks, some key nongovernment players felt that they were left outside. A health emergency, such as a pandemic, brings the public health system into direct contact with the clinical care system. For various reasons, this connection was not made as well as might be hoped. There can be various reasons for this. To begin with, it is widely acknowledged that the public health system, and the more entrepreneurially-based clinical care system, usually operate in separate worlds, and the communication between the two is often relatively weak (Tilson and Berkowitz 2006: 903). Furthermore, the clinical care system, particularly frontline physicians, have not developed the extensive networks more common among public health practitioners, and are usually not well represented in public health networks. Whatever the cause, the connection to this community was often not made well during the H1N1 events, with the result that many clinical physicians felt "out of the loop" and had to struggle to keep up to date with developments (Interview #8: January 15, 2010).

Conclusion

What we have seen in the post-SARS reports, and in some of the more recent commentary around the H1N1 pandemic, is a fairly typical reaction to emergency events. As stated earlier, disasters and fear of disasters generate a strong desire for hierarchy – somebody to take charge, or possibly someone to hold accountable (Waugh and Streib 2006: 131). As discussed, much of the post-SARS material falls in this category, with the partial exception of the *Naylor Report*, and even here there is a clear call for what we have called institutional simplification to deal with public health emergencies.

For the reasons discussed in this chapter, there are real disadvantages to resorting to a command-and-control model of governance to deal with public health emergencies. A more fruitful approach is to build on the networks that function between crises. The prevention of infectious disease, and the response to public health emergencies, can then be understood as exercises in network governance. It may well be that networks operating in times of crisis need to be more centralized than what is required in "peace-times," taking on the characteristics of what some have called "action networks" (Agranoff 2007: 10). Nevertheless, they can be understood as a form of network governance as adapted to the particular circumstances in play.

What, then, is the advantage of conceptualizing in this way public health governance during an emergency? The most obvious advantage is to resist the impulse to resort to command-and-control measures to deal with crises and to recognize that crisis operations "are multiorganizational, transjurisdictional, polycentric response networks" which "demand lateral coordination, not top-down command and control" (Boin and 't Hart 2003: 547). Failure to understand the network element of emergency response could mean under-estimating both the necessity and the challenges of involving a large number of autonomous or semi-autonomous actors, and developing the culture, the tools and the competencies to do so.

More specifically, an understanding of emergency response as a function of network governance adds clarity about the skills required for those directly involved in responding to emergencies. This particularly relates to the incident commander/manager, who will need to create shared norms, build and maintain commitment to the network, negotiate agreements, mediate in cases of conflicts between organizations and individuals, and, perhaps most important, build and maintain relations of trust among responders (Moynihan 2009: 13; Waugh and Streib 2006: 132). None of these skills seems implied in calls for a public health 'czar' or a 'commander-in-chief,' but are fundamental to the functioning of an effective network. In brief, the incident commander needs to understand his/her role as a network manager.

CHAPTER 5

GOVERNANCE IN 'PEACE-TIME': THE CASE OF THE CANADIAN HEART HEALTH INITIATIVE

Introduction

The previous chapter examined public health governance in 'war-time,' specifically crises relating to infectious disease outbreaks. But as stated earlier, public health plays in a wide range of different theatres. Although pandemics are much more likely to grab headlines, a great deal of work within public health goes to health promotion, and the prevention, management and control of chronic diseases, which claim many more victims in Canada than do infectious diseases. While similar language is used in both contexts – for example, in references to 'epidemics' of obesity or diabetes – the strategies to deal with chronic disease prevention differ considerably from what is done to respond to an infectious disease emergency. What, then, are the governance challenges in those circumstances, and how do they relate to network governance?

This chapter will look at the experience of the Canadian Heart Health Initiative (CHHI). The CHHI was probably not explicitly seen as an application of the network governance model by those leading the initiative. However, it was obviously conceived by individuals who saw the importance of collaboration in seeking to improve heart health in Canada. The CHHI represents an innovative attempt to bridge many of the fault lines discussed in chapter 1 which characterize the public health policy environment in Canada. In particular, it sought to construct a mechanism that would bring together governments – federal, provincial and local governments – and the voluntary sector in a partnership-based initiative. The fact that it had a twenty-year span in which it produced several important accomplishments demonstrates that many of its practices were successful and can possibly be emulated in other exercises. The fact that it was terminated before achieving its major objectives, on the other hand, suggests that it also contained some weaknesses to be avoided in the future. As will be discussed, perhaps the major weakness of the CHHI, from a governance perspective, was its failure or unwillingness to recognize that its largely horizontal approach existed within "the shadow of hierarchy" (Scharf 1994), and to find ways to successfully reconcile the two models.

There are, of course, many examples of experiments of health promotion and chronic disease prevention that can and should be examined from a governance perspective. The CHHI was selected for three main reasons. First, it is noteworthy because of its multi-level and multi-modal approach, as mentioned above. Second, its relatively long (twenty-year) history and the fact that, at its peak, it involved hundreds of organizations, governmental and non-governmental, make it stand out in the sector. Finally, the ability to examine an initiative in retrospect offers significant advantages, as it allows the observer to follow the CHHI through all of its various stages from beginning to end. In addition, key informants can view the initiative with more objectivity than might have been the case if the initiative was on-going.

Analytical framework

How, then, should the CHHI be examined? A number of frameworks have been proposed in the literature on collaborative governance, policy networks, network governance and related concepts, many of which were developed to apply to a specific case or cases. The challenge is to apply a conceptual lens that is general enough to encompass the various manifestations of collaborative governance, without being cast at such a high level of abstraction as to become difficult to apply to real world cases. For this, the framework provided by Ansell and Gash is useful (Ansell and Gash 2008: 550). After studying numerous cases, across several policy sectors, in the US and in many other counties, the authors propose a framework containing four broad categories of variables: starting conditions, institutional design, collaborative process and facilitative leadership. Each of the above categories is very broad and needs to be disaggregated further, but at the same time each presents a 'lens' through which to examine cases of collaborative governance, including network governance, and extract key issues. We will take each of these categories in turn, briefly discuss their significance drawing from pertinent scholarly literature, and seek to apply them to CHHI. The categories will be used as general guidelines, to be applied flexibly. In some cases, we will adjust the categories to take into consideration factors that are either missing or underemphasized in Ansell and Gash. In particular, we will adjust the framework to underline the non-linear relationship of the factors and to take better account of the federal reality of Canada. The framework, amended from Ansell and Gash, is represented below in Figure 4.

FIGURE 4: **Analytical Framework for CHHI**

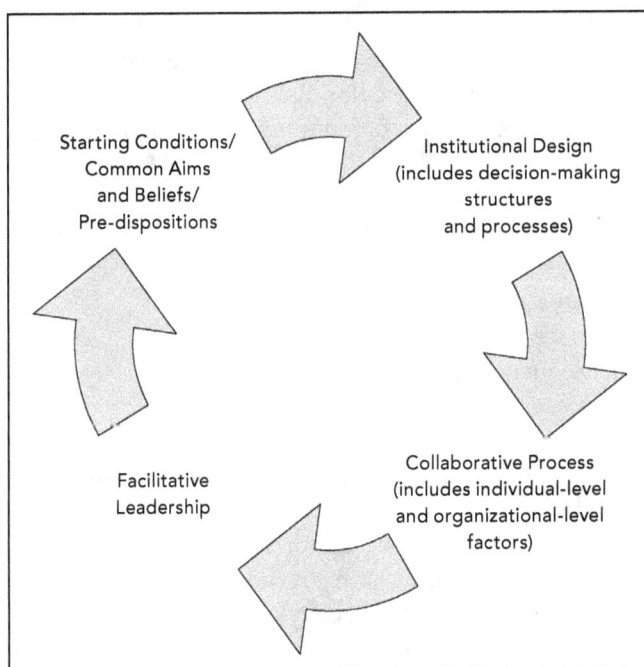

The methodology followed for the examination of the CHHI was a review of the published literature, followed by a series of semi-structured interviews with key informants. The process evaluation of the demonstration phase, prepared by the Conference of Investigators of Heart Health, was particularly useful for our purposes (Health Canada 2002). The interviewees were key players from the federal government, provincial governments, voluntary sector organizations and universities who had been directly involved in the initiative from the early stages and were, therefore, in a position to share important information and insights.

The Canadian Heart Health Initiative

The CHHI was initiated in 1986 in the wake of a paper produced for federal/provincial/territorial deputy ministers of health entitled *Promoting Heart Health in Canada* (Health and Welfare Canada 1987). It was designed "as a strategic linkage model employing coalitions to achieve partnerships and collaboration within and across sectors, and across national, provincial and local levels" (Health Canada 2002:4). Its long-term health goals were to:
- improve the heart health of Canadians;
- reduce premature cardiovascular morbidity and mortality;
- reduce the prevalence of preventable or controllable risk factors for cardio-vascular disease (CVD);
- improve lifestyle behaviours associated with heart health; and
- improve working conditions, social and physical environments supportive of citizens in making heart-healthy behavioural choices.

Its short-term health goals were to:
- increase public knowledge and awareness of the causes and consequences of CVD; and
- increase the knowledge and awareness of individuals at risk about how to control their CVD risk.

In addition, the CHHI established health system goals, which were to:
- maintain the provincial heart health programs and coalitions;
- entrench the issue of heart health into the agenda of governments and civil society organizations at all levels;
- disseminate the knowledge gained through the demonstration phase; and
- employ a public health approach to deliver integrated heart health programs.

A multi-level approach was taken for the CHHI, involving; the federal government, through Health Canada, all provincial governments,[16] and local communities. It followed a 'cascading'

[16] Territorial governments did not participate.

model in which broad directions were set at the national level; provincial-level coalitions were struck to coordinate activities in the province in question; and projects were carried out at either the provincial or local level. There was also an important international dimension, as representatives of the CHHI participated in international conferences to share information about the initiative (at that time Canada was seen as a world leader in the area of health promotion), and to learn from what other states were doing. Furthermore, the CHHI followed a partnership approach, in which it included voluntary sector organizations at all levels, as well as some private sector organizations such as media outlets. The various levels of the CHHI and the respective roles of the partners have been represented as follows:

International level:

- experiences from other countries drawn from; and
- contributions to major international heart health conferences.

Government of Canada (Health Canada) role:

- provided initial funding – matched by provincial governments;
- developed criteria for demonstration phase;
- provided technical assistance and secretariat support;
- organized workshops;
- established the Conference of Principal Investigators of Heart Health; and
- provided for the development, maintenance and dissemination of a national database.

Provincial role:

- Conducted heart health risk factor surveys;
- Assigned a responsibility centre to oversee planning and management of the demonstration phase, usually located within the provincial ministry of health;
- developed individual plans outlining specific goals and objectives for all projects; terms and conditions for coalitions and demonstration projects; theoretical foundations for interventions in the form of strategic plans or logic models; plans for recruiting partners for coalitions and projects activities.

Community-level role:

- designed projects to meet local needs (consistent with national criteria, and provincial terms and conditions);
- 259 demonstration projects in over 150 communities;
- each project supported by a multi-disciplinary, inter-sectoral team.

Voluntary sector/NGO role:

- Heart and Stroke Foundation served as the major non-governmental partner at the national level;
- provincial Heart and Stroke Foundation chapters acted as key non-governmental participants at the provincial level;
- several voluntary sector and other NGO partners involved at the community level, along with university researchers and private sector bodies, such as media organizations (Ibid.: 6-7).

Initial funding was provided by Health Canada, primarily out of the National Health Research and Development Program (NHRDP), and supplemented by discretionary funding. There was a requirement for matching funding by the province which was reflected in bilateral agreements on a province by province basis. In addition, there were in-kind contributions from NGOs and the private sector.

There were five distinct but overlapping phases of the CHHI:

1. Policy development, in which the broad lines of the initiative were developed;
2. Provincial heart health risk factor surveys, to assess scientifically the circumstances in each jurisdiction;
3. Demonstration phase, in which hundreds of projects at the local and provincial levels were launched;
4. Evaluation of the demonstration projects; and
5. Dissemination of results to the broader community (Ibid.: 9-10).

Unfortunately, there has been no evaluation of the initiative as a whole. However, a process evaluation was carried out on the demonstration phase, which is seen as the 'backbone' of the initiative (Ibid.: 10). From this we know that the initiative spawned 311 projects in all, amounting to a total expenditure of $36 million. Of the six strategies that were eligible to be funded under this initiative (public education, community mobilization, healthy public policy, strengthening preventive health services, research and evaluation, public health system leadership), 60 percent of the projects and 62 percent of the expenditures were on public education projects mostly related to modifiable risk behaviours (Ibid.: 17). The next most frequently used strategy, community mobilization, accounted for 17 percent of the projects.

The CHHI ended in 2006, when funding at the federal level was not renewed. (By this time, NHRDP no longer existed, having been absorbed within the Canadian Institutes for Health Research). The initiative can point to a long list of accomplishments, including provincial heart health risk factor surveys, several scientific papers on subjects related to heart health, and many community coalitions that continue to exist to this day. Perhaps its most significant achievement, as one of the key players of the CHHI put it, was "to change the discourse in Canada from heart disease to heart health," and through international meetings on heart health such as the one in Victoria, BC, in 1992, to change "the discourse on a global scale" (private correspondence with the author, April 28, 2009). However, the initiative must be judged as a partial success for two main reasons. First, it did not reach the deployment stage, as planned (Riley et al. 2009: I-21). Since the first five phases could be seen as building blocks towards an implementation strategy, not reaching this phase is significant. Second, and closely related to the first point, the overall health system goal of fully integrating heart health into the public health infrastructure was not realized (Health Canada 2002: 40). As will be discussed below, governance factors were an important determinant of the CHHI not completing its mission.

Starting conditions

Ansell and Gash indicate starting conditions "set the basic level of trust, conflict, and social capital that become resources or liabilities during collaboration" (Ansell and Gash 2008: 550). Some authors have referred to a similar notion as "predisposition" (Elliott et al. 1998: 607). Included in this are relevant issues such as a previous history of conflict or collaboration among the players. The existence of incentives, such as the possibility of accessing funding, is also often a strong motivator. Perhaps even more fundamental in setting the stage for collaboration is the existence of a common goal and a common set of beliefs. There must be what one observer has called "common…, agreed or clear sets of aims as a starting point in collaboration" (Huxham

2003: 404). This is key as an initial motivator, as well as the "bond" that holds a coalition together once it is established (Sabatier and Jenkins-Smith 1999: 122). Organizations seeking to act in concert with others will almost inevitably encounter differences in corporate culture, internal priorities, ways of operating and the like. Having at least a core base of commonly-held aims or beliefs can be a very potent force in overcoming the problems that come to the surface (Schlager 1995: 264). As will be discussed in chapter 9, it is important to be realistic about what one can expect in this area. It is not likely that partners will be in complete agreement on all aspects of the network's mission. Rather, what one should be seeking is a "minimum agreement which allows for joint action" (Termeer and Koppenjan 1997: 87). Furthermore, the recognition of the mutual interdependence of the players to achieve these aims is a critical part of starting conditions (Innes and Booher 2003: 40; see also Butterfoss et al. 1993: 320). Finally, the common aims and beliefs of the players in collaboration should not be seen as static. Although, as Sabatier and Jenkins-Smith have argued, core beliefs will be resistant to change, it is to be expected that what they call "secondary" beliefs, as well as the aims of the collaboration, will adjust as the collaboration advances and generates policy learnings.

As applied to the CHHI, there is good reason to believe that the holding of common beliefs and aims was one of the key factors in bringing the players together. 1986, the year of the initiation of CHHI, was a major turning point in the evolution of public health in general, and health promotion in particular, in Canada and internationally. This was the year of the *Ottawa Charter on Health Promotion*, a WHO initiative which signalled a new approach to health promotion. This approach was committed to dealing more directly with the determinants of health, which saw health in broad terms as "physical, mental and social well-being," and as a consequence of public policies both outside and inside the health sector (*Ottawa Charter for Health Promotion* 1986). Furthermore, at about the same time, "Achieving Health for All" was released, often called the *Epp Report* after the minister of health of that time, reflecting a similar approach as the WHO document and applying these principles to the Canadian context. (Epp 1987). The focus on a population approach to prevention of disease, community-level interventions, and partnerships is seen as signalling a new approach to public health (Riley et al. 2003:

754). These developments signalled a major shift in thinking in the area of public health in Canada (Stachenko 2001: 470).

It was in this environment that the CHHI was conceived. It was initiated by a small number of public health professionals in Health Canada and provincial governments who believed in the principles of the *Ottawa Charter* and the *Epp Report* and sought ways to translate these principles into practical reality (Interview #39: April 2009). *Promoting Heart Health in Canada,* the previously mentioned report developed for federal/provincial/territorial deputy ministers of health, reflected this approach and became the framework for the initiative (Health and Welfare Canada 1987). There were undoubtedly other incentives for participants to join this collaboration, probably the chief one being the possibility of accessing federal funding. But this does not appear to have been the major factor. The national consultation exercise which took place in the early stage confirmed a "broad national consensus… on the goals and strategies" of the CHHI (Health Canada 1992: 3). Moreover, the key informants interviewed stressed that the leading actors from the federal and provincial governments, as one put it, "were of like mind" about what was to be accomplished and how (Interview #38: April 2009).

More needs to be learned about the extent to which this set of beliefs penetrated all levels of the CHHI and whether it was maintained throughout its existence. However, from all indications, this was more than simply a "coalition of convenience." It was a collaboration in which the leading players, and the broader public health community, were united by a shared belief in both the goal and the methods in achieving that goal.

Institutional design

Ansell and Gash describe "institutional design" as "the basic ground rules under which collaboration takes place" (Ansell and Gash 2008: 550). There are many issues that can be considered in this context, such as frequency of meetings, optimum numbers of players, the existence or absence of dedicated support staff, the role of the chair, and so on. All are important issues which need to be taken seriously. In this review, however, we will attempt to focus on the more 'macro' issues: What are the structures for decision making? Who are the players involved and what mandates have they been given? And what are the power relations within the group? Questions related to funding will also be included in this discussion, since these formed a critical part of the decision making of the CHHI. How the intergovernmental relations were managed for this initiative will also be included in this section, since it was a critical factor in the institutional structure.

From the literature on the governance of networks, there appears to be no ideal model that will work best in all cases. Which model or style will be most effective will depend a great deal on a number of contextual factors (Mitchell and Shortell 2000). Certain key points emerge, however. The importance of inclusiveness is highlighted, not just for tactical reasons, but also because of the need for "collective, interactive discourse" (Hajer and Wagenaar 2003: 23). Transparency and fairness are also seen as important. A related question is the perceptions of power imbalances within the collaboration. Participants need to feel that they are being treated fairly, that there is a level playing field, and that they have a role in determining the broad directions of the network (Vangen and Huxham 2003: 21; Ansell and Gash 2008: 551). The need for good communication is also critically important (Butterfoss et al. 2003: 324), as is flexibility, to ensure the ability to make adjustments to changing players and circumstances (Lasker et al. 2001: 194).

Particular attention is given to the question of funding. There are several aspects to this question. The first is the question of the availability of funding, the importance of which is fairly obvious. Also significant is the question of the funding source – does it come from only one of the parties, or from more than one source? Multiple relationships will tend to 'equalize' power and set up more constructive relationships, whereas reliance on only one source for funding could create some dependencies that have a negative impact (Mitchell and Shortell 2000: 262). There is also the question of short-term versus longer term funding, which can also have an impact of internal dynamics. Mitchell and Shortell, among others, make the point that short-term funding can have a detrimental impact on partnership stability and sustainability (Ibid.: 254).

Also important is the question of how to accommodate the involvement of different orders of government in a collaboration. As mentioned earlier, the participation of two orders of government in collaboration creates an additional level of complexity to what is already a complex undertaking. Mark Imperial makes the useful point that different types of collaboration can coexist within a single policy network (Imperial

2005: 284). It seems fair to assume that the greater the complexity of the network, the greater the likelihood that this will occur. In this context, multi-level collaborations would seem more likely to encompass different types of collaboration, perhaps to the point of having networks within networks. As discussed earlier (chapter 2) in relation to the role of governments in network governance, it seems reasonable to posit, for example, that in a federal system of government, intergovernmental partners relate with each other in a way which is different from their interactions with other members of the coalition.

In Canada, because of overlapping jurisdictions in public health, mechanisms are necessary to manage federal/provincial/ territorial relations within the collaboration in this domain. However, as discussed in chapter 1, federal/provincial/territorial relations can operate at different levels within the same policy context. Johns, O'Reilly and Inwood have made an important distinction between 'intergovernmental relations' (IGR), which operates at the more strategic level and is usually handled by central agencies, and 'intergovernmental management' (IGM), which is carried out by the program areas in government. As Johns et al. have demonstrated, IGR and IGM may not share the same agendas and, in many cases, IGR officials may feel that those involved at the program level are too inclined to collaborate with their counterparts (Johns et al. 2006). This dynamic is apparently not unique to Canada; the same observation has been made with respect to other federations, such as Australia (Painter 2001: 140). We will return to this issue in our discussion of the CHHI.

The first point that is striking about the CHHI from an institutional design perspective is its lack of mandate at the federal level, and its lack of sanction from a federal/provincial/ territorial perspective. The Health Canada officials who were involved with the initiative did not see the need – and indeed deliberately avoided – seeking policy authority for the CHHI through a memorandum to Cabinet (MC) (Interview #38: April 2009; Interview #39: April 2009). They may have felt that their mandate could be drawn from the National Health Research and Development Program (NHRDP), but in actual fact, the CHHI was far more than a research program. Whatever the reason, the practical consequence of this was that Health Canada officials were participating in CHHI without a specific mandate to do so, and outside of formal scrutiny from within the federal government. This was compounded by the fact that the CHHI did not report to an established federal/provincial/territorial committee. At that time, an elaborate federal/provincial/territorial structure was in place in the health sector, in which intergovernmental committees and processes normally (but not always) reported to a federal/provincial/territorial committee at the deputy minister and/or the minister level.[17] In this case, the CHHI functioned outside the "orbit" of this committee structure, and therefore without the sanction or scrutiny of a senior federal/provincial/territorial forum (Interview #5: March 3, 2009; Interview #39: April 2009). Using Johns et al.'s useful distinction, therefore, this is clearly a case where intergovernmental relationships were handled at the program level, not the strategic level. Although the initiative began with an federal/provincial/territorial deputy ministers' working group, the CHHI was not established as part of a federal/provincial/territorial agreement or formal process. As a result, it would have been largely invisible to those dealing with intergovernmental relations at the more strategic level (Interview #5: March 3, 2009; Interview #38: April 2009; Interview #39: April 2009).

Consistent with its nature as a collaboration, the CHHI's decision making was consensus based, decentralized, and flexible (Interview #38: April 2009; Interview #41: April 16, 2009). The primary governance was established, not by an overarching framework agreement, but rather by a series of bilateral agreements between the Health Canada and individual provinces. The agreements were negotiated on a staggered basis, starting with Nova Scotia, followed by each of the other provinces at a time of their choosing. The agreement, developed collaboratively by Health Canada and the province in question, was then submitted to the NHRDP, housed within Health Canada. The agreements were drafted as research projects for the purpose of developing knowledge about interventions at the community level related to heart health. Once received by NHRDP, they were sent for peer review to ensure the scientific validity of the methodology. When approved, funding was made available, with the condition that this funding be matched by the relevant provincial government. A level of consistency was achieved by the fact that once the first

---

[17] This structure preceded the establishment of the Public Health Network, discussed in chapter 3.

proposal was reviewed and approved, it was used as a model for agreements with the other provinces.

At the national level, the CHHI was led by the Conference of Principal Investigators of Heart Health, which met at least annually. This committee did not seek to oversee what was taking place at the provincial level; rather, its function was primarily to establish the science behind the CHHI, discuss what additional knowledge products were needed, and strategize about next steps (Interview #38: April 2009). Working groups were created and studies were commissioned on a range of topics related to heart health. Beyond this, a forum called the Canadian Heart Health Network would be called once or twice a year to provide an opportunity for information sharing and skills development.

From an intergovernmental perspective, the relationships seem both collegial and science-based. In fact, the CHHI, particularly at the senior level, is an excellent example of a network housed largely within the same epistemic community. The program leads for Health Canada and for provincial governments were health professionals, usually chief medical officers of health. This provided a common language for the participants to use. It might fairly be said that the usual federal-provincial diplomacy was supplanted by scientific and technical issues that formed a common base for the discussion and for the relationships between the lead players (Interview #39: April 2009). The fact that the CHHI was characterized as a research initiative would have reinforced this tendency.

Notwithstanding the collegial nature of the relationships, there were power differentials within the CHHI. In the first instance, Health Canada took a leadership role through its access to funding. This enabled Health Canada officials to set the parameters around the funding, and therefore the initiative as a whole. It also appears that Health Canada officials provided a good deal of the intellectual leadership for the initiative. Neither of these factors seemed to have caused any apparent intergovernmental friction. On the contrary, Health Canada's leadership was welcomed (Interview #5: March 3, 2009; Interview #38: April 2009; Interview #41: April 16, 2009).

More fundamentally, there was an important power imbalance between governments and the non-governmental sector. The Heart and Stroke Foundation of Canada was identified as a national partner, but clearly it did not have the same role in the collaboration as a government. The power differentials were likely even greater at the provincial and local levels. The fact that federal and provincial governments provided most of the funding for the demonstration projects would have put them in a stronger position than voluntary sector organizations (VSOs), whose role was more related to delivery than to direction setting. This is somewhat at variance with the literature that calls for players in collaboration to be on a "level playing field." However, power imbalances are often very difficult to avoid, particularly when governments are involved (Nelson 2001: 93). In Laurence O'Toole's terms, networks "must combine the vertical elements of hierarchy and the horizontal components of functionally induced interdependence" (O'Toole 1997: 49). In view of these power imbalances, the CHHI might be seen as a sort of collaborative governance 'hybrid.' If so, it is probably in good company. As Innes and Booher have observed, collaborative governance in its "pure" form, happens only rarely, if at all (Innes and Booher 2003: 59).

The decision-making structures at the provincial level were both flexible and highly variable. By the terms of the funding agreements mentioned above, each province was required to form at least one coalition to carry out the demonstration projects. Eight of these operated at the provincial level, 33 at the local level. The composition and functioning of these coalitions differed from one case to another, and in some instances, their roles evolved as the process matured (Health Canada 2002: 12).

From this review of the CHHI's institutional design, the following conclusions can be drawn:

- the CHHI was established on a weak mandate, particularly at the federal level;
- intergovernmental relations were handled in a collegial, program-orientated and technically-focussed manner, outside of the orbit of more strategic intergovernmental discussions and relationships;
- it used a flexible, decentralized and consensual governance style;
- at its core, it was led by an 'epistemic community'; and
- while power imbalances were present, this did not seem undermine the CHHI's effectiveness as a collaboration.

What these elements meant to the eventual success or lack of it of the CHHI will be discussed in the conclusion of this chapter.

Collaborative process

The collaborative process variables go beyond the structural features of a network to ask what makes the collaboration work. These factors can operate at both the level of individuals and of the organization. As discussed earlier (chapter 2), at the individual level, there is a considerable emphasis in the literature on the importance of trust and, particularly, trust building among the players of a coalition (Imperial 2005: 304). Other factors which have been identified relate to the importance of direct communications, the effect of intermediate outcomes to provide some short-term movement to a process, and the cultivation of shared understandings of the initiative through mission statements and strategic plans (Ansell and Gash 2008: 550).

At the organizational level, participants in a network or coalition need to find a balance between their needs as an organization, and the role they play as a partner (Huxham and Vangen 2000: 1170). Network members, particularly voluntary sector organizations, in the first instance, must still strive to ensure their survival as an organization (Provan and Milward 2001: 420). How this balance is struck is a central issue. An important concept in this context is congruence between the objectives of the individual organization and the objectives of the coalition. In an ideal world, the organization, by pursuing the needs of the coalition will be pursuing simultaneously their own organizational objectives. A VSO which champions, say, cancer prevention, may be very supportive of an initiative which addresses modifiable risk factors relating to heart health, because cancer and CVD share many of the same risk factors (tobacco use, physical inactivity and unhealthy eating). At the same time, however, that agency depends on fundraising, and will likely want to avoid losing its visibility in an initiative which is based on another disease group, or even an initiative that is more generic in seeking to address common risk factors. Unfortunately, there appears to be little research on this issue (Sabatier and Jenkins-Smith 1999: 138), and questions remain about what might be the 'tipping point' in an VSO's willingness to support an initiative which might be aligned with its objectives, but may run contrary to its need to survive.

There are a range of other issues which operate at both the individual and the organizational levels. For instance, it is not necessarily clear how the players maintain their level of commitment as the collaboration evolves. As discussed earlier, at least a minimal level of shared aims and beliefs is fundamental to collaboration. However, shared beliefs alone may not be sufficient to sustain a coalition when it almost inevitably runs into challenging issues (Elliott et al. 1998: 618). As participation in a coalition is usually voluntary for the participating individuals and organizations, the benefits of participating must outweigh the costs for players to stay on board (Butterfoss et al. 1993). What these factors are will undoubtedly vary greatly depending on individual circumstances.

Certain key issues emerged from the CHHI. At the interpersonal level, trust certainly appears to be one of those factors. As previously stated, the CHHI was initially brought about by a relatively small group of like-minded individuals who knew each other from previous capacities. As medical officers of health, they shared a common training and understandings, and approaches. Key informants also pointed out that while the leaders were strategically placed within federal and provincial governments, their involvement was driven by their personal and professional interest and commitment to public health, rather than by the formal positions they occupied within their respective organizations (Interview #38: April 2009; Interview #39: April 2009). Indeed, because they were for the most part below the level of deputy minister, a part of their role was to advocate within their respective organizations for support, including financial support.

Another factor which was important was the achievement of 'intermediate outcomes.' The phased-approach of the CHHI might well have built in a sense of momentum and provided encouragement for the players to carry on. The fact that the first two phases – to set the overall policy direction and to conduct the heart health risk factor surveys – were conducted fairly quickly likely contributed a sense of positive movement. Several scientific reports from working groups assigned to various issues were also produced at different stages. Finally, the demonstration phase was focussed on projects, primarily at the local level, which would have given a tangible sense that the initiative was producing outputs and therefore helped to fuel the process.

At the inter-organizational level, the picture appears more complex. As we have seen, the intergovernmental relationships do not seem to have been problematic. What is not clear is how the voluntary sector organizations (VSOs) balanced their own organizational interests with those of the CHHI. At the national level, since the Heart and Stroke Foundation of Canada was the 'lead' VSO, and the initiative was about heart health, one can infer a considerable amount of congruence.

What took place at the community level is much less clear. Both the process evaluation of the demonstration phase and the situational analysis (Riley and Feltracco 2002: v) refer to "turf wars" having been a significant liability throughout the CHHI. This was also confirmed through interviews, although one key informant suggested that the conflicts may have been more of a problem in the earlier stages of the initiative (Interview #42: February 2009; Interview #43: February 2009). Unfortunately, what is lacking is a clear picture of what was behind these conflicts. From the information we have, it seems that these conflicts were primarily at the community level during the demonstration phase. Indeed, an initiative like this one, involving as it did hundreds of organizations, is bound to experience instances of internal conflict. There is some indication that the tension was between VSOs, as well as between the national, provincial, and local chapters within certain VSOs (Interview #42: February 2009). However, a much more intensive scrutiny would be necessary before any firm conclusions could be made. What can be asserted is the absence of mechanisms to deal with these conflicts when they arose. Training was available in different forms in different communities, including in conflict resolution, group management and team-building. In some cases, facilitators were provided to the projects (Health Canada 2002: 36). More broadly, however, there is no evidence of a deliberate, consistent approach to the management of conflict when it arose.

With respect to the factors related to the collaborative process, therefore, the CHHI presents a multi-faceted picture. On the one hand, among the leaders of the initiative, one can observe strong interpersonal relationships among individuals who shared common beliefs and a common professional training. There were also a number of intermediate outcomes in the form of surveys, reports, studies and projects that would have served to give encouragement to the participants and a sense of momentum. The duration of the initiative for a twenty-year period is an indication in itself that the collaboration was functional. At the same time, the existence of internal 'turf wars' is indicative that there were weaknesses within the collaborative process. This may have been the result, as one interviewee indicated, of lack of clarity, or differences in perception about roles and responsibilities (Interview #42: February 2009). It could also be due to inadequate internal communications, conflicts about funding issues, interpersonal conflicts, or a combination of some or all of these. What can be said is that the lack of a consistent and effective mechanism to deal with these internal conflicts was potentially damaging to the initiative's effectiveness and sustainability.

Facilitative leadership

As discussed in chapter 2, the importance of leadership and, particularly, a certain style of leadership, is an important determinant to the success of a network. Roussos and Fawcett, for example, found that in studies on partnerships, leadership was the most often reported internal factor (Roussos and Fawcett 2000: 385). It seems clear that every coalition will need champions – sometimes called policy entrepreneurs, or policy brokers – to help define and articulate its mission and to seize opportunities that arise on the policy landscape (Khator and Brunson 2001: 156; Kingdon 2003). Furthermore, given the nature of a collaborative venture, the style of leadership needs to be of the 'facilitative' nature. As many of the partners will see themselves as equals, a rigid hierarchical model is not appropriate. This will be particularly the case in a network involving different orders of government, each sovereign within its own jurisdiction. This style of leadership is well-captured by Roussos and Fawcett in saying that it is "a process of persuasion or example by means of which an individual (or leadership team) induces a group to pursue objectives held by the leader or shared by his or her followers." (Roussos and Fawcett 2000: 385). Paquet goes further, and argues that modern governance requires "stewardship" rather than "leadership" (Paquet 2008). While the style of leadership more typical of collaboration is somewhat 'gentler' in comparison to the command-and-control model, it nevertheless demands a high level of tenacity and single-mindedness to ensure the collaboration holds together and moves forward in achieving its goals. Huxham refers to this balance by saying that leaders of collaborations have to operate from a spirit of collaboration and what he calls "collaborative thuggery" (Huxham 2003: 417).

Scholars have made the important observation that collaborations generally evolve over time, and that the type of leadership needed will change as the coalition matures (Roussos and Fawcett 2000: 385). Butterfoss has suggested four stages in a collaboration: formation, implementation, maintenance and accomplishment of goals or outcomes (Butterfoss et al. 1993: 322). What might be needed at the formation stage to provide a vision and mission may not be the same skills that are needed at the implementation or maintenance stages. Whereas policy entrepreneurs might be needed for the first phase, given their ability to recognize and seize opportunities and take personal risks, it is likely that the needs will shift more to policy managers in the more mature phases. The skills of the latter will be given to sustaining the coalition and adapting as necessary to adjust to changing circumstances (Takahashi and Smutny 2002: 168). Takahashi and Smutny go so far as to say that coalitions may contain the "seeds of longer-term partnership failure" if they do not adjust to these changing leadership needs (Ibid.: 180).

Good leadership appears to have been one of the CHHI's great strengths and, perhaps, from a long-term perspective, one of its major weaknesses. From the published material, confirmed through interviews, it is apparent that the leadership for the initiative was concentrated in a small group of individuals and with one individual in particular, emerging as the central figure. Throughout its evolution, the leadership of the initiative at the national level revolved primarily around Dr. Andres Petrasovits, described by Riley and Feltracco as the "linchpin" of the CHHI (Riley and Feltracco 2002: 10). This characterization was repeatedly emphasized both in the written material and in the key informant interviews (Interview #38: April 2009; Interview #39: April 2009; Interview #41: April 16, 2009; Interview #43: February 2009). From all evidence, the leadership style of the initiative was more 'charismatic'[18] in the Weberian sense, than bureaucratic, and appears to have remained so for its entire duration. Moreover, there is little to suggest a shift towards a more managerial style as the initiative evolved. Although the commitment of Dr. Petrasovits and his colleagues is evident, the CHHI does not

---

[18] One of the interviewees emphasized that Dr. Petrasovits was not charismatic in the traditional sense, in that he tended to be rather modest and unassuming, but nevertheless was "the one who kept the thing going" (Interview #41: April 16, 2009).

appear to have been 'institutionalized' within Health Canada, which left it vulnerable when changes of personnel or priorities occurred within the department. It is perhaps indicative that the demise of the initiative generally coincided with Dr. Petrasovits' unfortunate death. Other factors were perhaps more significant in understanding the demise of the CHHI, in particular the termination of the NHRDP, the primary federal funding source, as well as the increased interest in 'integrated' as opposed to single-disease health promotion strategies (Interview #5: March 3, 2009; Interview #38: April 2009; Interview #39: April 2009). Although it would be difficult to weigh the relative importance of these factors, the lack of a transition from a charismatic style of leadership to a more bureaucratic style appears quite significant.

Unquestionably, the leadership of the CHHI went beyond this small group of individuals at the national level. Leadership was needed at the provincial level for the risk factor surveys, and to establish and maintain the provincial and sub-provincial coalitions in the demonstration phase, as well as the evaluation and dissemination phases. Given the large number of projects that were initiated as part of the CHHI, this also suggests quite a diverse pattern of leadership styles applied in a wide range of circumstances. What this pattern was, and what leadership styles emerged at the provincial and local levels, are questions that cannot be addressed here.

Conclusion

Our opening proposition was that factors related to collaborative governance played a major role in the CHHI's not being able to achieve some of its key objectives. This is not to argue that the CHHI was a failure. On many scales, it made a very important contribution to the field of heart health, and health promotion in general. It was an experiment that was closely monitored, and sometimes emulated by other countries. At the broadest level, it changed the discourse from a cardio-vascular disease model to a health promotion model, in Canada and eventually globally. Specifically, it commissioned several studies and reports that were very useful in their time and which are still pertinent today. On the ground, some of the 'demonstration' projects proved themselves to be sustainable, and remain in place. Finally, the CHHI established a platform on which future health promotion strategies could build. For example, some have argued that the Pan-Canadian Healthy Living Strategy, launched in 2005, could be considered part of the legacy of the CHHI (Riley et al. 2009: I-24).

The CHHI demonstrated some innovative ways of bridging the fault lines in public health described in chapter 1. In the first instance, it was clearly effective in overcoming the intergovernmental divisions so common in Canadian public policy issues. On the basis of the process evaluation supported by interviews with key informants, there is no indication of federal/provincial/territorial tensions being played out within the initiative. On the contrary, the provincial representatives were satisfied with their roles in the initiative, and were supportive of the role played by the federal government. Provincial governments, for their part, were also able to cement effective partnerships with local governments. Second, effective partnerships were forged between governments at all levels, and VSOs. Admittedly, at the local level, VSOs were active primarily in the service delivery function, rather than playing a meaningful role in policy development. However, at the national level, the Heart and Stroke Foundation of Canada was at the central table and participated in shaping the initiative along with federal and provincial governments.

Admittedly, the CHHI was less successful in bridging the third fault line discussed earlier, that relating to the intersectoral divide. A part of this can be attributed to the fact that its leadership was part of the same epistemic community, which made it easier for the principals to communicate with each other, but probably more difficult to communicate with others who were not part of this community. In fairness, however, the CHHI was focussed primarily on the health sector, and reaching out to a broader community was not a major priority.

The most significant factor for the CHHI's premature demise was its failure to reconcile the horizontal and vertical axes of governance. Most fundamentally, it tried to function in the absence of sanction and a formal mandate. This was a two-sided coin. On the one hand, it meant the CHHI could operate free of constraints, which provided an opportunity for flexibility, innovation and experimentation. Furthermore, the fact that it was outside the 'strategic' intergovernmental relations discussions allowed it to avoid becoming entangled in the fairly acrimonious federal/provincial/territorial disputes in the 1990's relating to funding for health care. It might even be questioned whether the initiative would have been launched if it had sought formal federal/provincial/territorial sanction, which was precisely the fear of the originators (Interview #39: April 2009). On the other hand, the lack of sanction and mandate also meant that the initiative could easily be ignored or forgotten. When the funding source on which it drew ended in 2002, there was no formal agreement or mechanism on which to base a case for its continuation, and no champions for it around the federal/provincial/territorial deputy ministers' table (Interview #39: April 2009). There was no formal decision to end the CHHI, because there had been no formal decision to initiate it. The consequence was that it ended "with a whimper, not a bang." As one informant stated: "It just kind of died" (Interview #38: April 2009).

Indeed, integrating the vertical and horizontal dimensions of governance is one of the most daunting challenges of network governance. How to accomplish this is likely to be very context-specific. The fact that the CHHI was able to function for as long as it was may be a testimony to the fact that public health – perhaps more than most sectors – can be receptive to non-hierarchical approaches. This is particularly the case in areas such as health promotion and prevention of chronic diseases, which require a long-term perspective. Notwithstanding the use of such terms as the obesity 'epidemic,' these areas are less likely to be perceived and responded to as public health emergencies. Nevertheless, an initiative such as the CHHI, which does not reconcile its need to function collaboratively with the fact that it functions within a hierarchical bureaucratic structure, may enjoy some short-term successes, but is not likely to prove sustainable in the longer term.

III – EXPANDING THE BASE

CHAPTER 6

THE VOLUNTARY SECTOR IN PUBLIC HEALTH GOVERNANCE: PARTNERS IN NAME ONLY?

Introduction

We have previously discussed the role – or, more accurately, the lack of it – of voluntary sector organizations (VSOs) in the public health network (PHN) (chapter 3). However, the role, potential or real, of VSOs extends far beyond the PHN. Indeed, the voluntary sector is quite pivotal in public health. Unfortunately, no reliable estimate is available of how many organizations are involved in the various dimensions of public health. However, given the length and breadth and diversity of the sector, it is safe to assume that they constitute quite an impressive number.[19] More than simply a question of numbers, however, is the role they play. Public health departments and agencies at the national, provincial and local level often rely on VSOs to reach vulnerable clients at the community level. In addition, there exists a myriad of organizations playing an advocacy role on a full range of issues, including mental health, infectious diseases, chronic diseases and injury prevention. In this way, they provide a "window" into the interests and concerns of the community of interest. VSOs can also be repositories of considerable expertise, often playing a major role in research in such areas as heart disease, cancer and mental health.

---

[19] In the health field as a whole, it is estimated that there are approximately 5,300 voluntary sector organizations (VSOs) that are directly involved (Imagine Canada 2007b).

The purpose of this chapter will be to discuss the place of the voluntary sector in public health governance in Canada. Is their role, as it is currently played out, consistent with the network governance model? The chapter will begin with a brief overview of the voluntary sector in general, as well as its place in Canada, and more specifically in the national public health arena. Following this, a typology will be proposed of the various types of relationships between VSOs in the public health sector with government at the national level, providing examples of each type of relationship for purposes of illustration. The chapter concludes with a discussion of what the current configuration means for the prospects of network governance in the public health sector in Canada. Our general proposition is that while the voluntary sector has a key role to play in the governance of the public health area, much of this potential remains untapped, and that while there are a few recent examples which appear to 'break the mould,' it is far from clear whether these should be seen as aberrations or as indications of new directions for the future.

The voluntary sector: Terminology and context

A number of different terms can be found in the literature related to this sector, with overlapping but not identical meanings which can lead to a certain amount of terminological confusion. Civil society, non-governmental organizations, non-profit organizations, the 'third' sector, philanthropic organizations, and interest groups are all fairly common terms, but do not always carry the same meaning. Civil society is often understood to mean "the broad range of social institutions that occupy the social space between the market and the state" (Salamon et al. 1999: 3) but this can sometimes be understood to include both for-profit and not-for-profit organizations. In the same way, 'non-governmental organization' can also include both types of organizations. In this chapter, we will use the term 'voluntary sector,' which we take to mean all organizations led by boards, the members of which serve on a voluntary basis. This does not mean that these organizations are composed entirely of volunteers, as in many cases they have salaried personnel to carry out their activities. Moreover, these are organizations which operate on a not-for-profit basis for the purpose of achieving a public good. Finally, they are understood to be formally independent from government, even though, as will be discussed, they may work quite closely with government, or may indeed receive a significant portion (if not all) of their funding from government.[20] Using 'voluntary sector' rather than non-profit or not-for-profit has the added advantage, as has been pointed out by others, of avoiding describing the sector in the negative, that is, as not being something else (Phillips 2001: 259 fn. 3).

The importance of the voluntary sector is not new in liberal democracies. Indeed, de Tocqueville attached a great deal of importance to this sector as a "necessary guarantee against the tyranny of the majority" (de Tocqueville 1945: 201-202). Freedom of association also features prominently in the First Amendment of the US Constitution, which is sometimes referred to as the *Magna Carta* of the voluntary sector in that country. More recently, it has been quite common in American literature to cite the importance of the "Iron Triangle" in public decision making: the three points of the triangle being congressional committees, the bureaucracy and "interest groups" (Pross 1986: 97).

Since the 1960s, the role of the voluntary sector, consistent with the notion of modern governance, has undergone a fairly significant transformation. A. Paul Pross observed that the diffusion of power in modern society "has transformed participating interest groups from useful adjuncts of agencies into vitally important allies" (Ibid.: 243). Indeed, VSOs are now often the delivery agents for government programs and services, and are increasingly finding a place in the development of research and public policy (Brock 2001: 263; Juillet et al. 2001: 25). The increasing importance of the voluntary sector is evidenced in the fact that in the late 1990s, both the UK and Canada produced major reports on the role of the voluntary sector, followed by "compacts" (in the case of England and Scotland) and an Accord (in the case of Canada) to guide relations between government and the voluntary sector (United Kingdom 1998; Privy Council Office 2001).

Notwithstanding the above, there can be a high level of diversity in the nature of the relationships between government and the voluntary sector across different policy sectors of the same government (Coleman and Skogstad 1990: 25; Boris and Steuerle 1999: 14-15; Salamon 1999: 330). What is true in agriculture, for example, may or may not resemble what takes place in human

[20] This definition is consistent with that used in *Building on Strength: Improving Governance and Accountability in Canada's Voluntary Sector (Broadbent Report)* 1999: 7; see also Morison 2000: 98.

resource development, or in the cultural sector. One can often
see a considerable amount of diversity even within the same
policy sector (Coleman and Skogstad 1990: 29). This diversity,
combined with the fact that this area has been relatively under-
studied, means any generalization must be approached with
caution. Still, the area is too important to overlook, given the
centrality of the voluntary sector to our subject. As Stoker puts
it: "The governance perspective demands that these voluntary
sector, third-force organizations be recognized for the scale and
scope of their contribution to tackling collective concerns without
reliance on the formal resources of government" (Stoker 1998: 21).
Focusing our discussion on the area of public health will help to
narrow the range of circumstances to some degree, but even here,
the relationships between government and VSOs can be highly
variable and complex.

Susan Phillips has provided a useful framework for an
analysis of government-voluntary sector relationships – and one
consistent with the notion of network governance – by suggesting
that increasingly, governments must make a shift from governing
by programming to governing by relationship-building. As
Phillips points out:

> The primary responsibilities of government in relationship
> building are to provide an appropriate enabling environment
> to permit the partners to fulfill its [sic] potential, to ensure
> that government commitments on particular standards of
> conduct can be met by relevant departments, and to facilitate
> collaboration, including means for reviewing and improving
> the relationship.

Phillips goes on to argue for the need to shift "from traditional
programming that focuses on hierarchy, accountability, and
funding within a single department to relationship building that
involves collaboration, coordination, responsiveness, and flexible
accountability..." (Phillips 2001: 258). Taylor expresses a similar
notion in referring to the transition from a "contract culture to a
partnership culture" (Taylor 1997: 21).

For our purposes, we need to ask how close the public health
sector is to making that shift.

The voluntary sector in Canada

To begin, it is necessary to situate the public health voluntary
sector in the context of the broader voluntary sector in Canada,

since that is the environment in which the former must function. In comparison to many other countries, Canada's voluntary sector is quite robust, at least in terms of the number of organizations in existence, and the number of individuals involved. Based on a survey conducted in 2000 by Johns-Hopkins University and Imagine Canada, the share of the voluntary sector workforce (paid staff and volunteers) in the economically active workforce in Canada is second only to the Netherlands (Hall et al. 2005: 9). Imagine Canada estimates that in 2008, the voluntary sector generated $106.4 billion in economic activity, or 7.1 percent of Canada's GDP (Imagine Canada 2011). This study also found that the number of people involved in the voluntary sector in Canada was particularly high in the health and housing sectors (Hall et al. 2005: 13).

At the same time, however, the voluntary sector in Canada has faced some serious challenges in the past decades. From about the mid-1990s, the sector came under significant scrutiny, in part because of issues raised by John Bryden, a Liberal Party MP from Ontario. Mr. Bryden asked a number of challenging questions about the accountability, transparency and representativeness of a number of organizations the government was funding (Miller 1998). To deal with the controversy surrounding the issue, Finance Minister Paul Martin Jr., initiated a review of the funding of 'interest groups' in 1994. Concurrent with these developments, the federal government entered an intensive deficit-cutting exercise initiated in the 1995 federal budget. For the voluntary sector, this meant that there would be considerably less funding available. This dealt a severe blow to the sector which, since the 1960s, had become heavily dependent on government funding (Ibid.: 408). Many VSOs had to absorb severe cuts to their budgets, and in some cases, funding was terminated altogether. This also meant the continuation and, probably acceleration, of a trend away from operational funding, sometimes called 'core funding,' in favour of project funding (Phillips and Levasseur 2004: 453). Combined with this was a tendency in favour of contracts and contribution agreements of short duration, instead of the multi-year arrangements that had previously been more common (Ibid.: 457). The scarcity of funding meant that the competition for funding among VSOs became that much more intense (Imagine Canada 2007b: 8), and that these organizations had to account more rigorously for the money they received.

Faced with the challenges described above, it is probably not an exaggeration to describe the voluntary sector in the mid to late 1990s as being in crisis (Miller 1998). Since the larger VSOs could still depend on outside revenue streams, the impact of these developments was more significantly felt by small and mid-sized organizations. Still, the sector as a whole felt under pressure, and was searching for a way to establish itself on a stronger foundation.

Recognizing that there were important issues that needed to be addressed, the voluntary sector established the Voluntary Sector Roundtable (VSR) in 1995 to discuss the challenges faced by the sector. In 1997, the VSR initiated a panel, under the leadership of former NDP leader Ed Broadbent, to examine how to improve accountability and governance in the sector, and how to improve the sector's relationship with the federal government. The panel produced a final report titled *Building on Strength: Improving Governance and Accountability in the Voluntary Sector,* which was tabled in 1999. Among the 41 recommendations of this report was the creation of a joint federal government-voluntary sector task force to address the issues facing the voluntary sector.

Parallel to this, in 1998 the federal government created the Voluntary Sector Task Force (VSTR) for the purpose of developing a joint agenda and action plan. This was structured as a collaborative process with three joint tables which together produced a joint report called *Working Together.* This report formed the basis of the Voluntary Sector Initiative (VSI).

The VSI, which functioned from 2000 to 2005, was a $94.6 million joint initiative between the federal government and the voluntary sector to attempt to address some of the issues facing the voluntary sector. Its objectives were to improve the relationship between the two parties, build sector capacity in the areas of finance, human resources, policy and knowledge and information management, and improve the regulatory and legal framework under which the sector operates (*Voluntary Sector Initiative Impact Evaluation* 2009: xi). The VSI had a number of positive accomplishments over its five-year term, including improved statistical information about the voluntary sector; recommendations on regulatory reform (although only a small number were actually implemented); an awareness campaign; policy internships and fellowships; a National Learning

Initiative; and a number of tools, manuals and best practice information (Hall et al. 2005: 24).

The major outputs which had the potential of altering this relationship were *An Accord Between the Government of Canada and the Voluntary Sector,* and two "codes of good practice," one dealing with policy dialogue and the other with funding. The accord was a high-level statement of principles which borrowed heavily from the compacts developed in the UK (Brock 2004: 170). The policy code was to provide guidelines for "open, informed, and sustained dialogue" between the voluntary sector and the government, while the funding code was to help guide interactions on funding policies and practices. Also of key importance from the perspective of engaging the voluntary sector in policy discussions with government was the sectoral involvement in departmental policy development (SIDPD). This program, which accounted for 30 percent of the total VSI budget, was to enhance opportunities in federal departments for policy input from VSOs, and to strengthen the capacity of VSOs to input into governmental policy-making exercises.

Notwithstanding the short-term accomplishments, it does not appear that the VSI had a long-term, or even medium-term, impact in changing the relationship between the voluntary sector and the government. The *Voluntary Sector Initiative Impact Evaluation,* produced by Human Resources and Skills Development Canada, concluded that the accord and the codes are not currently "living documents" and that they "neither guide nor improve the relationship between the federal government and the Sector or improve the capacity of the Sector in any significant or systematic way" (*Voluntary Sector Initiative Impact Evaluation* 2009: 14). The same evaluation concluded that there is limited evidence that SIDPD projects had "any impact on increasing the mutual understanding of the government and voluntary sector" (Ibid.: 34). The two elements of the VSI that were deemed sustainable were the Human Resources Council and the Satellite Account, both of which are research and survey-based initiatives (Ibid.: 57). Indeed, the evaluation implicitly raises a question about the commitment of government at the time to 'true' collaboration when it states that: "In terms of opportunities for policy input and true collaboration, a desire on the part of government is necessary and should be in place if another VSI-like initiative is undertaken" (Ibid.: 52).

The federal government has acknowledged that "the VSI suffered goal overload and was unrealistic in its scope" (Ibid.: xii). At the end of the initiative, it put in place the voluntary sector strategy (VSS), a four-year, $12 million program to complete the remaining elements of the VSI, which included conducting the impact evaluation.

Unfortunately, the VSI's work was made more difficult by the 'crisis' in grants and contributions at what was then Human Resources and Development Canada (HRDC) in 2000. The controversy was precipitated by an audit on management controls which suggested that many grants and contributions in that department had not been properly accounted for. The government response to these events was to impose a number of additional requirements on VSOs about how they must account for the monies they received (Phillips and Levasseur 2004: 451; Gibson et al. 2008: 413). These requirements added significantly to the administrative load of organizations at a time when they were already dealing with staff cuts and insecure funding.

That the challenges for the voluntary sector continued following the VSI is evidenced by the report of the Independent Blue Ribbon Panel on Grant and Contribution programs. This panel reported in 2006 that many voluntary sector organizations "are in a fragile state, hostage to costly funding delays and to reporting requirements that many are ill-equipped to meet" (Blue Ribbon Panel 2006: 13). Although the language of "partnerships" is frequently used, "in most cases, the government has the weight and the authority to impose terms and conditions on its funding partners that they are hardly in a position to resist" (Ibid.: 2). Indeed, the Blue Ribbon Panel remarked that the uncertainty and instability affecting the voluntary sector was worse than ever (Ibid.: 7). In their submission to the panel, the Canadian Council on Social Development (CCSD) wrote that: "Non-profits are being treated by government in a fashion that reflects a lack of faith in their trustworthiness and competence..." (Ibid.: 15). The same conclusion has been arrived at by Phillips and Levasseur (2004) and Gibson et al. (2008). Moreover, many of the *Broadbent Report*'s more far-reaching recommendations, such as establishing a voluntary sector commission, identifying a Cabinet minister to articulate the concerns of the sector at the Cabinet table, and assisting voluntary sector organizations to develop the capacity for improved public reporting, still have not been implemented, and there is no evidence to suggest that they are even under consideration.

Returning to Phillips' criteria, it would seem that governance based on relationship-building is still a long way off. The observations of the Blue Ribbon Panel and the CCSD, and even the impact evaluation, suggest nothing like "an enabling environment to permit partners to fulfill [their] potential..." Furthermore, no enforcement monitoring mechanism has been put in place "to ensure that government commitments on particular standards of conduct can be met by relevant departments..." The conclusion that the Voluntary Sector Accord, the policy code and the funding code are not currently "living documents" makes this all the more clear. Moreover, there is no longer a mechanism in place "to review and improve the relationship..." (Phillips 2001: 258). Finally, the "flexible accountability" posited by Phillips as a characteristic of governance by relation-building has not come to fruition. Indeed, as discussed, the governmental response to the HRDC events of 2000 has led to even more stringent requirements on funding arrangements with VSOs. Describing the effects of the accountability regime in place for VSOs as "overwhelmingly negative" for that sector, Phillips and Levasseur argue: "Above all, it is hurting the relationship between the federal government and voluntary organizations in significant ways because there is a considerable loss of trust" (Phillips and Levasseur 2004: 464). More generally, the previously referenced report on the voluntary sector by Hall and his colleagues identifies a lack of a coherent policy framework related to the voluntary sector in Canada, and cites this absence as "one of the biggest constraints to its future development" (Hall et al. 2005: v).

The difficult climate for VSOs reflects a major power imbalance between these organizations and governments (Phillips and Graham 2000: 171). Project funding rather than core funding, short-term funding arrangements rather than multi-year funding, and an inflexible accountability regime all suggest a desire by government for control in the relationship with the voluntary sector. From a policy perspective, VSOs are often relegated to the position of the "attentive public," rather than as a "sub-government," that is, as strong players in the policy process (Pross 1986: 149). The consequence of this is that they find themselves at the consumer end of public policy, rather than being in a position to have a significant role in shaping policy. While common in Canada, as will be seen, this is not the only type of relationship between government and VSOs that is feasible or even appropriate. There are many international examples that can be drawn in which VSOs have a direct role in the public policy process, in some cases going so far as to include the ability to veto state proposals (Salamon 1999: 353). On the other hand, the power imbalances in government-voluntary sector relationships are not conducive to building trust between partners, which is consistently identified in the literature as a crucial element of network governance. The consequence is the perpetuation of a relationship with government that in many respects fails to live up to its potential.

What makes the public health voluntary sector special?

The state of the relationship between the federal government and the voluntary sector sets the context for relationships with the public health sector. Referring to period of deficit-cutting in the 1990s, Colin McMillan, president of the Canadian Medical Association, and Seema Nagpal, pointed out that the "weakening of the partnerships between government and the voluntary sector [...] tended to undermine efforts to develop public health programs based on the concepts of the Lalonde and Epp reports" (McMillan and Nagpal 2007: 62). What distinguishes public health somewhat from many other sectors is two-fold: the multiplicity and diversity of VSOs involved in public health, and the role of advocacy in the activities of these organizations and in public health in general.

As noted earlier, the voluntary sector is particularly active in the health field. It has been estimated that health sector organizations comprise 31 percent of the total workforce of the voluntary sector (Brock et al. 2007: 10). This relationship has deep roots. Chapter 1 referred to the creation in 1919 by the federal government of the Dominion Council of Health (DCH). In what may be seen as an early step in the direction of collaborative governance, the DCH was composed of the deputy minister of health, the provincial chief medical officers of health, as well as representatives of organized labour, women's groups, social service agencies, agriculture and universities (Rutty and Sullivan 2010: 2.19). The purpose of the body was to advise the newly established federal Department of Health, and there is some indication that the DCH was in some ways "more important to the development of public health during the 1920s than the fledgling department it served" (Ibid.:

3.1). The Canadian Red Cross also played a major role, funding its own public health programs, and providing salaries for public health nurses to supplement what provincial governments, such as the one in Ontario, were providing (Ibid.: 3.3). In the area of emergency response, for instance, both the St. John Ambulance and the Canadian Red Cross were heavily involved in efforts to contain the 1918 influenza pandemic and, in fact, are typically involved in most major crisis situations.

In more contemporary times, the diversity of public heath has inevitably led to a wide range of VSOs involved in one of the many aspects of public health. Organizations might be engaged in preventing infectious disease such as avian flu, the West Nile virus, HIV/AIDS; behaviour-based strategies, such as smoking-cessation, alcoholism, unsafe sex, family violence, use of personal communication devices in automobiles, promoting physical activity, healthy eating habits, and sun safety; life-stage related issues related to children and seniors; gender-based concerns, most often related to women's health, including maternal health; planning for emergency response; generic chronic disease prevention and control as well as disease specific activities (cancer, heart, lung etc.); settings-based strategies (school, work, communities, etc.); and groups taking a determinants of health approach, which tend to focus on poverty, housing and social justice. There are also a number of professional associations of physicians, nurses, dietitians, physical therapists, psychologists and others which play an active role in the field. The end result is that it is very challenging for governments to determine with whom to collaborate and how, and for the organizations themselves to know which players are involved in the issues that affect them.

Another significant factor which characterizes government/ VSO relationships is the centrality of the advocacy function in public health. The question of whether VSOs can be partners with governments and advocates for their 'cause' at the same time can be a major source of tension (Young 1999: 59). This tension, therefore, is not unique to public health. Yet it has a particular saliency in that sector (Chapman 2001: 1226). Public health practitioners, whether employed by governments, VSOs, or in private practice, see one of their roles as advocating for the types of changes in society that will lead to improved health of the population (see J.M. Last's definition of public health in chapter 1). This may lead to a greater willingness for public health agencies to enter into partnerships with VSOs to achieve shared objectives, leading to the multiplicity of relationships mentioned above. It can also lead to unorthodox, but not necessarily unusual, situations in which government representatives work alongside VSOs in campaigns to pressure their own governments to make particular changes to an area of public policy that affects health.

Three types of government-VSO relationships

From the above, it follows that the nature of the relationships between the voluntary sector and government is fraught with complexity. Some of the key questions to be answered include:

- Are VSOs in public health involved substantively in public policy issues, or is their role restricted to being simply delivery agents?
- How significant and pervasive is the power imbalance between governments and VSOs, and to what extent does it hinder more effective relationships?
- Are there instances where governments relinquish their leadership role to become simply 'one of the team,' and if so, what are the circumstances which allow this to happen?
- Are there appropriate mechanisms in place to allow for effective dialogue between government and VSOs?
- What is the appropriate place for advocacy in these relationships?

As a first step toward answering these questions, it is necessary to distinguish the types of relationships that exist in the sector. For this we will use Dennis R. Young's typology of state/voluntary sector relationships at the national level in the US (Young 1999: 33). Young proposes these relationships be divided into three broad categories. What he calls the "adversarial model" is one where the main objective of the VSO is to pressure government to make public policy changes it considers necessary or advisable. These have often been called "pressure groups" or "lobby groups" (see for example Pross 1986). What he calls the "complementary model" is one where VSOs – he uses the term "non-profit organizations" – are seen as extensions of government, in that they deliver programs and services financed by governments according to criteria and conditions established by government. Finally, the "supplementary model," is one where the VSO "fulfills demands for a public good left unsatisfied by government." In this case, the VSO fills a gap that the state either cannot or will not fill itself.

Interestingly, Young's typology corresponds quite closely to the one proposed by Coleman and Skogstad some years earlier to describe different types of policy networks: pressure pluralism (adversarial model), state-directed networks (complementary model), and clientele pluralism (roughly, supplementary model) (Coleman and Skogstad 1990: 26-30).[21] We will draw from both in applying these three categories to the public health sector in Canada.

The adversarial model

In this instance, the ultimate objective of the VSO is to influence public policy in a way to advance its particular cause.[22] Whether by choice or necessity, it is not dependant on the state agency (at the national level, either the Public Health Agency of Canada or Health Canada) for financial support or other resources. This financial independence frees it from "the 'whims and rules' of the funding agency" (Grieve 2003: 117), although it could also mean that the organization pays a high price for its 'freedom,' in that it lacks the resources to be effective in advancing its cause. While the state agency cannot control this type of VSO, it may well be sympathetic to its objectives and at times even lend some form of 'moral' support. In some instances, representatives of the state agencies may participate in processes led by the VSO, which can lead to situations, where the representative of the state agency participates in an endeavour that seeks to influence public policy, thereby conflating the public health advocacy role with that of public servant. We include in this category VSOs which receive no funding or direct assistance from PHAC or Health Canada, as well as the larger VSOs who may receive some support from those agencies, but whose funding base is so large and diverse (including from different sources within the federal government) that this support does not put them in

---

[21] Two other categories proposed by Coleman and Skogstad, "parentela pluralism" and "closed systems," are not applicable because, in the first case, the category does not apply to the national level, and in the second, the public health environment is too fragmented to operate as a closed system.

[22] The use of the term 'adversarial' can be misleading, since, as will be seen below, the relationship with the government agency can be positive as well as negative.

a position of dependence. On the other hand, the relationship inherent in the adversarial model is such that it tends to put considerable distance between the VSO and the public policy development process, thus relegating those organizations to the position of the 'attentive public,' as opposed to a more substantive 'sub-government' role.

Without attempting to claim that these are necessarily 'representative' – a claim that would need to be substantiated by a comprehensive study of VSOs in the public health sector, which is beyond the scope of this book – the examples below are meant to illustrate these types of relationships. The information provided is based on a literature review, supplemented by interviews with key informants as noted.

Prevention of Violence Canada

Prevention of Violence Canada (POVC) is a network composed of a range of stakeholders which include governments at the local, regional, provincial/territorial, and to a lesser extent, federal levels, provincial and territorial public health associations, other voluntary sector organizations, research organizations, individual university researchers and private sector parties. Although its roots go back to the mid-1990s with a position paper by the Canadian Public Health Association (CPHA) titled *Violence in Society: A Public Health Perspective,* it was initiated by a resolution at the 1998 Ontario Public Health Association annual meeting to create a violence prevention workgroup with a view of raising consciousness about the importance of violence prevention as a public health issue. Since operating at the provincial level was felt to be inadequate, the initiative was then raised to the national level through a resolution passed by the Canadian Public Health Association in 2004. What emerged was a coalition of members which met through town hall meetings, often as part of CPHA's annual conference, the first being held in 2005. There were also a series of meetings of the steering committee, as well as six workgroups, which met primarily through teleconferences and email. Although the goals of the initiative varied somewhat over the years, the Fifth Annual Town Hall meeting (2009) identified its goals as: developing a national violence prevention strategy for Canada; garnering support for a public health approach to violence prevention; putting violence prevention at the same level of priority as law enforcement; and developing a methodology to measure results (Prevention of Violence Canada 2009). There is no dedicated secretariat and the co-chairs take their role on a rotational basis. POVC actively draws from the international community, adopting the WHO *Preventing Violence: A Guide to Implementing the Recommendations of the World Report on Violence and Health* as the framework for the national violence prevention strategy (Ibid.).

POVC is an advocacy organization; it does not seek a programmatic role for itself. The funding it seeks to support violence prevention, largely from the Public Health Agency of Canada, is intended for organizations working in the area, depending on the nature of the activity, rather than attempting to carry out the activities itself. Over the years, it has received small amounts of funding to allow it to stage a town hall meeting, to allow its members to travel to some international meetings, or to cover the costs of some teleconferences for its members. The level of funding received was not significant or regular enough to compromise its independence. However, the key informants interviewed felt quite distant from the government apparatus and the public policy-making decision-making process (Interview #16: July 12, 2010; Interview #46: July 20, 2010). Indeed, a good part of their advocacy work revolved around strengthening their relationship with the federal government agencies, so it could have a stronger role in the policy process as it relates to the prevention of violence (Interview #16: July 12, 2010).

Federal representatives, primarily from the Public Health Agency of Canada, have provided moral support to POVC, and at times have provided advice to POVC leaders on strategy and tactics, while at the same time abstaining from voting on initiatives, conscious of their ambivalent status. Representatives from provincial and territorial governments also participate in POVC discussions, which are less problematic for provincial/ territorial representatives, since the network primarily seeks to influence policy at the federal level.

Safe Communities Canada

Safe Communities Canada is a national VSO that was established with the objective of building capacity in communities across Canada to mount coordinated and collaborative injury prevention campaigns. Its core program is the Safe Community 'designation', by which it recognizes communities which are addressing injury prevention in an effective way. In addition, it also produces a 'National Report Card' which provides a national profile on injury prevention and individual community score cards by which those in the network of Canadian Safe Communities can measure their standing *vis-à-vis* the national profile. It is also active internationally as an accredited certifying centre for the WHO Collaborating Centre on Community Safety Promotion.

Historically, Safe Communities Canada has not received significant funding from the federal government. Its financial support derives essentially from three sources: project grants from provincial workers' safety boards (47 percent); contributions from the corporate sector (23 percent); and sales of products and tools to provincial agencies and foreign countries, such as Australia (30 percent). Although its main focus has been at the program level, Safe Communities Canada has come to the conclusion that it needs to have much more impact at the national policy level. As a result, it has recently entered into discussions with the three other major injury prevention VSOs – Safe Kids Canada, Smartrisk, and ThinkFirst Canada – to discuss the possibility of merging into a single organization. The motivation for this integration is precisely to be more effective at engaging the federal government in policy discussions, with the objective of establishing injury as a stand-alone health category, which the organizations believe is not now the case. The new organization would be expected to compete more effectively with other public health VSOs for the attention of federal government agencies, such as Health Canada and PHAC, including the opportunity to receive funding from those agencies. Ideally, the new organization would eventually find itself in a position of participating in joint planning and decision-making processes with the federal government.

Although Safe Communities Canada has maintained its independence from the federal government and, therefore, its ability to take the policy positions it considers appropriate, its formal relationship with that government is suboptimal (Interview #32: July 14, 2010). Specifically, its ability to enter into policy discussions is at best sporadic. The government's decision, announced in the March 2010 Speech from the Throne, to fund an national strategy on childhood injury prevention, while providing some modest funding to the organizations, has not led to any significant changes in the relationship between these groups and the federal government (Interview #33: March 2,

2011). The decision of the four injury prevention groups to even discuss seriously the possibility of merging into one can be seen as an eloquent expression of the perception of these organizations as being marginalized in the policy process. The possibility of integration with others is no doubt a painful decision for many in those organizations, implying as it does not only having to abandon their respective institutional 'brand,' but also that several staff positions would be affected, starting at the top, where three individuals would have to relinquish their positions as president in favour of the fourth. Although these efforts ultimately may not bear fruit, the incentive to seriously consider taking this step would need to be very powerful, demonstrating that for these groups, the *status quo ante* is seen as being unacceptable.

Centre for Science in the Public Interest

Perhaps the 'purest' example of the adversarial model is the Centre for Science in the Public Interest (CSPI). CSPI is a non-profit, health advocacy organization which conducts research and advocates for policy change in areas related to health and nutrition, and which seeks to provide consumers with useful health-related information (Interview #53: June 24, 2011; www.cspinet.org). The organization emphasizes that it is an independent body, which does not, and will not, receive funding from either government or industry. Instead, it derives its funding exclusively from revenue derived from the distribution of its newsletter, and donations from its list of subscribers. CSPI has been very active in pressing for public policy changes in a number of areas. From 1997 to 2003, its main focus was on mandatory nutrition labeling on food. Since then, it has expanded its focus to include sodium reduction, sugar reduction, advertizing aimed at children, food safety, and a number of other issues. Its approach to advocacy centres on "enlisting the support of intermediate decision makers," in particular other VSOs, print and broadcast media, public servants and political representatives (Interview #53: June 24, 2011).

While maintaining its independence from government, CSPI participates actively in various fora established by government, and is not reluctant to take public positions critical of the government when it feels this is warranted. For example, it is a regular participant in consultations by Health Canada on issues related to nutrition and participates actively on working groups to look at various aspects of food policy.

While CSPI welcomes opportunities to participate in joint planning or policy development exercises, as it did with the Sodium Working Group and the Trans-fat Task Force, it guards its independence carefully. A key informant from CSPI indicated that they would participate in such exercises only on the condition that they maintain the right to express a dissenting opinion if they disagreed with the majority view (Interview #53: June 24, 2011). CSPI sees most of its focus on pressing for public policy changes from the outside, and is wary about working too closely with government. The organization sometimes encounters difficulties enlisting the support of other public health VSOs for various advocacy campaigns, perhaps due to the concern of those organizations to maintain, or at least avoid damaging, their relationships with government (Ibid.).

To encapsulate, the above examples are meant to illustrate cases where the VSOs, whether by necessity or by choice, have remained independent from government, thus allowing them to take positions they consider appropriate. At the same time, those groups operate outside the formal public policy process, and have few tools to influence it, other than persuasion of government representatives, participating in consultations when they are held, or resorting to such devices as letter-writing campaigns or appeals through the media. While these organizations can become quite heavily involved in government consultation processes, such as CSPI's involvement in the Sodium Working Group, on the whole the relationship between these VSOs and government agencies, whether by necessity or by choice, is quite limited.

The complementary model

In the complementary model, the relationship between the state and the VSO is one in which there is a clear power imbalance, with the state being the dominant actor. As Phillips and Graham point out "...governments are often guilty of assuming that the weight of their dollars give them the authority to dictate accountability mechanisms and policy directions, rather than to negotiate them" (Phillips and Graham 2000: 180). Essentially, the state agency maintains its control, consciously or otherwise, through the use of financial transfers. With the federal government, this generally takes two forms: grants and contribution agreements.[23]

[23] We will not discuss government contracts, since that does not go beyond what is essentially a commercial relationship.

The former is meant to refer to transfers where there are fewer conditions and less onerous reporting requirements than in the case of contribution agreements. In reality, the two mechanisms often resemble each other, with more conditions attached to grants than might normally be expected (Blue Ribbon Panel 2006: 3). Although care is taken to avoid a principal-agent relationship in the strict sense, (see Salamon 1999: 349 for a discussion of this relationship), the funds are provided to a VSO as part of a policy or program objective the government wishes to pursue.

Because many VSOs in this situation essentially depend on government transfers to remain in existence, the priorities and original mandate of the organizations can easily become distorted as they pursue government funding opportunities (*Broadbent Report* 1999: 5). Over the long-term, this tends to diminish the independence of an organization that falls within this category, as it begins to resemble "a quasi-governmental entity" (O'Connell 1996: 224). In such instances, the VSO risks losing credibility in the eyes of other VSOs as well as with its own members (Pross 1986: 198; Interview #4: June 24, 2010; Interview #6: September 8, 2010). Somewhat paradoxically, such an unequal relationship can even limit the VSO's value to government. While more convenient for the state agency in the short-term, it also deprives its representatives of an opportunity to enter into a more fruitful policy dialogue which could be beneficial to both parties.

As stated earlier, the tendency of VSOs to be more tightly controlled by the state has probably increased since the mid-1990s. VSOs can be quite resilient and highly creative, even under pressure from reduced funding opportunities and additional accountability requirements. In many cases, they are often quite capable of finding ways to express their views on policy issues, directly or indirectly. Yet for those VSOs in this category, dependence on government funding remains an inescapable factor in shaping their relationship with government and, ultimately, to the broader VSO community. This is, in particular, the case with smaller organizations dependent primarily on one revenue source. Even in the case of the voluntary sector initiative (VSI), a joint federal government-voluntary sector intervention which was designed to reflect a spirit of partnership and horizontality, the accountability mechanisms in the contracting arrangements essentially undermined the collaborative aspect of the relationships (Phillips 2004: 13).

Examples of VSOs in the public health sector which fall in this category include the multitude of organizations receiving funding under the PHAC's community-based programs, such as the Community Action Program for Children (CAPC) and the Canada Pre-natal Nutrition Program (CPNP). CAPC and CPNP, which are PHAC's largest contribution programs by a considerable margin, with annual budgets of $55 million and $26 million respectively, are structured to involve consortia of local organizations to engage in a range of initiatives to improve the circumstances of at-risk children. Organizations involved might be hospitals, housing corporations, service organizations, professional associations, and many others. Large organizations can be involved, but the majority tend to be relatively small community organizations. Although a high percentage of these groups receive funding from other sources, the federal government funding is often seen as the centrepiece around which other funding is assembled (Interview #45: July 20, 2010). In many cases, without the funding from PHAC, they might cease to exist, or at least be forced to drastically curtail their operations. The same could be said for many organizations receiving funding from a number of other PHAC programs.

The point to be made is not that these organizations necessarily feel frustrated that they do not have a stronger role in the policy process. In many cases, their primary goal is to provide a service they consider important and beneficial, not to participate in policy discussions. In general, however, what these relationships reflect is a significant power imbalance in favour of the state. The fact that most of the funding agreements are of short duration – recently they have been held to one or two-year renewals – serves only to underscore the unbalanced nature of these relationships.

The supplementary model

As referenced earlier, Young describes this model as one where outside agencies perform a role or provide a service that the state agency either will not or cannot provide. In these cases, the level of the relationship is on a much more equal basis than is the case with the complementary model. The VSO may be dependent on the state agency for financial support, but at the same time, the state agency is dependent on the expertise that the VSO possesses. Entering into such relationships may be viewed as an admission by the state agency (sometimes grudgingly made) that it does not possess the knowledge or capacity to carry out a particular activity or strategy. In such cases, the role of the state agency is quite circumscribed, largely restricted to providing funding, and allowing the VSO a greater than usual amount of discretion with the use of that funding. Using the terminology described earlier, the VSO involved in such a relationship is acting more in terms of a "sub-government" than as a member of the 'attentive public.'

Interestingly, this type of relationship is both young and old in the health sector. In the early part of the 20th century, many health institutions in some provinces, such as tuberculosis sanatoria and hospices, were left to the private sector, particularly faith-based organizations, to administer (Rutty and Sullivan 2010: 3.7). Catholic and Anglican missionaries were also left to operate small hospitals in the North. Similarly, in the 1940s, the Canadian Red Cross provided many of the district nurses in remote areas (Wallace 1948: 175-176). Another example is the Canadian National Council for Combating Venereal Diseases (later renamed the Canadian Social Hygiene Council), a VSO which implemented venereal disease campaigns in most provinces and major cities (Rutty and Sullivan 2010: 3.10). As the municipal, provincial and federal governments developed and expanded their competencies, particularly following the Second World War, they asserted control over many of these services. The more modern manifestation of this model, however, provides an interesting and promising departure from the more conventional models. Two recent cases can be made to illustrate this point.

Canadian Partnership Against Cancer Corporation

The origins of the Canadian Partnership Against Cancer Corporation (CPACC) date from 1999, when four leading organizations decided to collaborate to develop a strategy against cancer. These organizations were: the Canadian Cancer Society; the National Cancer Institute of Canada; The Canadian Association of Provincial Cancer Agencies; and Health Canada. This collaboration, which also involved a large number of smaller cancer-related organizations in Canada, led to the development of the Canadian Strategy on Cancer Control (CSCC), which was formalized in 2006. A decision was made in that year by the Government of Canada, to provide funding ($287 million over 5 years) to the CPACC to implement the CSCC. CAPCC does not include a direct service delivery capacity, since this falls in the jurisdiction of provincial governments. Furthermore, it does not seek to address the entire cancer control universe.[24] Rather, the CSCC is a knowledge-based strategy whose purpose is to "maximize the development, translation, and transfer of knowledge and expertise across Canada" (*Canadian Strategy for Cancer Control* 2006: 4). The CSCC works on the basis of eight strategic priorities: primary prevention; screening/early detection; surveillance; development of evidence-based diagnostic and treatment standards; clinical practice guidelines; research; health human resources; and patient-centred support. Once the decision was made to fund the CSCC, CPACC incorporated as a non-profit organization, led by a board of directors of between 15 and 18 members, which include a broad constituency of VSOs, as well as federal (1 seat on the board) and provincial/territorial government representatives (5 seats on the board, in addition to Quebec, which has an *ex officio* representative).

The CPACC model is a major departure from either of the adversarial model or the complementary model. In his case study of CPACC, Michael Prince described the cancer strategy as "a platform for communication between governments, non-government agencies, health professionals, and cancer survivors and families" as well as "an opportunity to modernize the management of chronic diseases and to further democratize the conduct of intergovernmental relations" (Prince 2006: 468). In fact, CPACC's mandate goes well beyond this. CPACC is a case where the VSO, as a result of a decision made at Cabinet, has been given policy authority and financial resources to implement a national cancer prevention strategy (Interview #27: September 23, 2010; Interview #37: September 27, 2010). This may well be unprecedented in modern times in the health sector. In a sense, CPACC represents a case where the tables have been turned on the state parties. As a consequence, Health Canada and the Public Health Agency of Canada often find themselves in the position of participating, not as parties with a stronger role than any other organization, but as one of many parties. If either agency has a particular interest in one of the eight strategic priorities, or in a sub-strategy within them, it may decide to participate more actively by contributing funding for a particular purpose. This was the case recently when PHAC and Heart and Stroke Canada

---

[24] Where there are instances of joint interest, the CAPCC and organizations in the health portfolio (Health Canada and the Public Health Agency of Canada) have been instructed to ensure the actions of one informs the other.

contributed funding to CPACC for the Collaboration Linking Science and Action (CLASP) programs to integrate cancer and other chronic disease prevention programs. Because they were providing funding, both organizations received a seat at the table to participate in steering those programs.

Although funded by the federal government (primarily Health Canada) and reporting to the Minister of Health, CPACC clearly enjoys a great deal of autonomy. The fact that the government's funding commitment was over a five-year time horizon, and can be extended, further reinforces this level of autonomy. CPACC was also given the authority to provide funding to third parties, thus conducting its own calls for proposals, and the flexibility to reallocate funding across priorities, as it determines appropriate, both of which are highly unusual (Interview #37: September 27, 2010). Instead of a power imbalance in favour of the state agency, as in the other two categories, the establishment of CPACC represents an attempt to establish a different type of relationship. There has been some speculation about the motive behind the federal government's decision to establish and fund CPACC as it did. Prince suggests that the strategy may have been a response to public pressure for federal and provincial governments to work more closely together on cancer control and other health issues. He also suggests that the *Kirby Senate Committee Report* and the *Naylor Report*, as well as the report from the Romanow Commission, may have contributed by adding pressure to the calls for reforms to healthcare policy, delivery and governance in Canada (Prince 2006: 471). One can also speculate that because tens of thousands of Canadians regularly volunteer for cancer-related funding drives and other activities, political leaders may tend to be especially responsive to the objectives of cancer organizations. Beyond these more 'political' factors, CAPCC/CSCC also presented an opportunity to build from a knowledge base beyond what state agencies could offer. The fact that all three major political parties supported the CSCC in the 2006 election campaign suggests a view that the existing governmental apparatus, for whatever reason, was not capable of achieving the goals of a national cancer strategy. Whatever the motivations that led to it, the fact remains that what was created was a dramatically different model from what has typically been the case.

The Mental Health Commission of Canada

The Mental Health Commission of Canada (MHCC) is in some ways similar to CPACC, but its relationship with the federal government stops short of going to the same extent. MHCC stemmed from the recommendations of *Out of the Shadows at Last*, a voluminous report produced by the Senate Standing Committee on Social Affairs, Science and Technology, chaired by Senators Michael Kirby and Wilbert Keon. The recommendation to establish an arm's length commission to focus on mental health was accepted by the federal government, with the support of the provinces and territories. MHCC was established as a non-profit organization in 2007, with four major goals in mind: to act as a catalyst for reform of mental health policies; to act as a facilitator, enabler, and supporter for a national approach to mental health; to work to diminish the stigma and discrimination associated with mental illness; and to disseminate evidence on all aspects of mental health to governments, stakeholders and the public. It is funded over 10 years, with the possibility of renewal beyond that period.

Since its inception, MHCC has worked on developing a mental health strategy, which it is doing in two stages. In the first stage, it developed a framework for such a strategy, titled *Toward Recovery and Well-being,* which was released in November 2009. The second stage consists of developing a comprehensive strategic plan for how to achieve the framework. In addition, it is working on developing anti-stigma initiatives; conducting research demonstration projects on homelessness issues; engaging in knowledge exchanges; and developing a network of partners in the mental health area.

There are similarities between MHCC and CAPCC in that, in both cases, the government considered it necessary to go outside the formal bureaucracy to accomplish its objectives in these areas. More specifically, the government considered that it lacked the capacity, or was not strategically placed, to deal effectively with the issues of cancer prevention or mental health respectively. MHCC falls short of the CAPCC mandate in that it is charged only with developing a mental health strategy, and did not receive the policy authority or the funding to implement this strategy, although it is conceivable that this could be viewed as a next step. Furthermore, MHCC did not receive a mandate from Cabinet, but was established using the Prime Minister's prerogative (Interview #18: April 1, 2011). Still, it represents a departure from the more typical relationships represented by the 'adversarial' and 'complementary' categories. To begin with, its agreement with Health Canada is that it will not engage in advocacy, which differentiates it from 'adversarial' categories. While this can be seen as a restriction to its activities, it is more significant in underlining that rather than being on the outside advocating for changes, it is a central part of the public policy apparatus dealing with a difficult issue. In other words, it is not an outsider looking in, but rather the other way around.

Second, while it receives its 'core' budget from Health Canada, its ten-year mandate, as well as the latitude it has received to develop a framework and a strategy for mental health, does not reflect the same type of power imbalance as the organizations in the 'complementary' category. Similar to CPACC, it acts as a funding agent in its own right, providing funding to other VSOs in the mental health area. Furthermore, as with CPACC, government departments, such as PHAC and Human Resources and Skills Development Canada have provided funding to partner for specific projects, but in these cases, it is MHCC, and not the government department, that is the "senior partner." While not being as ground-breaking as in the former case, MCHH remains significant in that it establishes the basis for a different relationship between the state agency and the VSO. Perhaps the best indicator of the 'out of the box' nature of both CPACC and MHCC is that central agencies, such as the Treasury Board Secretariat, are reported to have expressed considerable concern and even discomfort about the terms for the establishment of both entities (Interview #18: April 1, 2011).

Hybrids

Categorizing the many relationships that exist in the public health sector runs the risk of oversimplifying what are often very complex situations. As Young acknowledges, the categories above should not be seen as mutually exclusive. Many combinations and permutations can and do exist in the 'real' world. We will look at just two such examples.

The Canadian Strategy on HIV/AIDS

Peter Tsais conducted a case study of the Canadian Strategy on HIV/AIDS during the 2000-04 period. At that time, five national VSOs formed a coalition for the purpose of delivering Health Canada's HIV/AIDS program. According to Tsasis, each organization committed itself to three main objectives: to strengthen community capacity in responding to HIV/AIDS; to forge coalitions and partnerships with key players within the community; and to develop strategic objectives, policies and plans related to people living with HIV/AIDS and vulnerable populations (Tsasis 2008: 267). Each organization was dependent on federal government funding, as that represented over 50 percent of the total budget of each organization.

The key aspect of Tsasis' article is to examine the power relationships between the VSOs and Health Canada. The author makes a convincing case that a significant power imbalance existed in that relationship, which was used by Health Canada to "exercise power in many integral facets of their activities" (Ibid.: 271). He goes on to say that the VSOs found their advocacy role curtailed by Health Canada's "formalization and bureaucratization" and that while Health Canada referred to the arrangement as a "partnership," from the perspectives of the VSO participants, the power imbalance inherent in the relationship made it a "pseudo partnership" (Ibid.: 273).

Tsasis goes on to show that over time, the VSOs were able to neutralize, to some extent at least, that imbalance by forging strong relationships between each other, and drawing on the social capital they had built as a result of their activities at the community level. In so doing, they were able to rebalance their relationship with Health Canada. Tsasis concludes from this that "a dependent organization can gain leverage over the dominant organization by co-opting actors who can constrain, through their influence, the actions of the dominant organization in a way that favours the dependent organization" (Ibid.: 285). In the end, however, although the VSOs were pushing back against Health Canada's dominance, their actions were essentially defensive in nature, and did not alter the fact that what was involved was at the core an 'us' and 'them' relationship, seemingly based on a lack of trust.

Canadian Breast Cancer Initiative

Malcolm Grieve's case study on the Canadian Breast Cancer Initiative provides an interesting example of supplementary and complementary models co-existing within the same policy community. In this case, Grieve sees a hierarchy in the networks that are involved in this issue. On one side are the members of an 'epistemic' community,[25] that is, professional organizations and research institutions which are involved in breast cancer, such as the Canadian Cancer Society, the National Cancer Institute of Canada, and the Medical Research Council (now the Canadian Institutes for Health Research). Grieve uses Coleman and Skogstad terminology to describe the relationship between these groups and Health Canada as an example of 'clientele pluralism,' in that they offer a resource knowledge, which the state can not easily provide itself (Grieve 2003: 105). This relationship is characterized by the presence of long-established groups from the medical profession which have a previously established relationship with government officials, in this case Health Canada. In many cases, they will have partnered in the allocation of funds, using methodologies, such as peer review panels, that are familiar and comfortable for them (Ibid.: 105).

On the other side are voluntary sector representatives, in particular those involved in the Canadian Breast Cancer Network. In contrast to the professional groups, Grieve describes the relationship in these cases as being more characteristic of the complementary model that is essentially acting as delivery agents for the state. Rather than being part of the 'sub-government,' as was the case with the professional organizations, these tend to be confined to the role of the 'attentive public,' whose main levers to influence policy is through the media (Ibid.: 105). What emerges from this is a complex picture where there are different levels of inclusion within the same policy community, between those who have a previously established relationship to government and those who must play on the margins. Based on the proliferation of groups, leading to further fragmentation of views and competition, without collaboration between them and a weakening relationship between the government and the Canadian Breast Cancer Network, Grieve sees reasons to doubt the long-term influence of the voluntary sector in this area (Ibid.: 120).

[25] See chapter 3 for a discussion on epistemic communities in public health.

Conclusion: A base to build on?

The picture of the relationships between the government and the voluntary sector in the public health field is thus a complex one. How does one put this in perspective and what does it this mean for the prospects for network governance? Recognizing that Phillips' model of governance by relationship building is still somewhat of an ideal-type, one can legitimately ask how far we have progressed down this road. Our conclusions will need to be tentative, in part because, as Klitgaard and Treverton have noted, "we are not even close to having a model to assess partnerships" (Klitgaard and Treverton 2004: 50). Still, some observations can be made, preliminary though they might be.

First, the adversarial model, as reflected in the cases reviewed, represents only a heavily circumscribed form of collaboration. In these instances, neither the state party nor the voluntary sector party is committed to working together, although this can change if the government agrees to provide tangible support for a particular initiative. Although there may at times be joint tables or fora, these will tend to be more informal or sporadic, unless the organization, as is the case with the CSPI, has an independent funding source. There is far less possibility that there will be an agreement on joint planning and activities. There may be participation of government officials in some discussions led by the VSO, as we have seen, but the conflict in roles will inhibit the full participation of the government representative. In this model, the VSO will be in the position of the "attentive public," with very few direct policy levers to effect policy change.

The complementary model, by which the state will attempt to achieve its policy objectives by using the voluntary sector as its delivery vehicle, is different from this in the sense that it is based on a formal relationship. The state agency and the VSO will have agreed to some common goals which the VSO will carry out with agency funding. The VSO, if it is creative, can enjoy a fair measure of autonomy, which from a legal liability perspective, the government will seek to encourage (Interview #26: September 23, 2010). Nevertheless, the fact remains that this is a relationship of dependency favouring the state party. The power imbalance implied from such a relationship is hardly conducive to trust building or collaboration.

CPACC, and to a somewhat less extent, MHCC, appear as the clearest examples of the supplementary model. Although funded primarily through the federal government, the VSO in these cases functions in a sub-government capacity, acting as a third-party funder while maintaining an arm's-length relationship with government. It is possible to argue that the CAPCC model, in particular, may simply have turned the complementary model on its head. Instead of the VSO party being the junior partner to government, with CAPCC it is now the VSO that is in the driver's seat with the state party confined to a secondary role. Interviews with key informants, however, suggest that the relationship appears to be evolving (Interview #37: September 27, 2010; Interview #27: September 23, 2010; Interview #48: June 10, 2010). Whereas in the first years, both parties seemed to be eager to keep each other at a significant distance, more recently some joint activities have been initiated, as with the CLASP initiative mentioned above. How the relationship will evolve still remains to be seen, as does the question of whether the government will choose to replicate this model. It does, nonetheless, create the potential for a qualitatively different type of relationship and one more consistent with modern governance than what conventionally has been the case. On the surface, at least, these seem considerably more consistent with Phillips' characterization of governance by relationship-building involving "collaboration, co-ordination, responsiveness, and flexible accountability."

Aside from these two cases, the overall picture that emerges regarding the relationship between the government at the national level, primarily the Public Health Agency of Canada and Health Canada, and the voluntary sector may be described as follows. First, what one finds is a pattern characterized by a high level of diversity and complexity, with a very large number of VSO players, and quite a number of different arrangements that have been negotiated over a long time horizon.

Second, there is an apparent lack of an overarching strategic approach or framework in either Health Canada or the Public Health Agency of Canada to guide arrangements with the voluntary sector. Rather, such relationships emerge on a case-by-case basis, according to the particular circumstances of the case. Some key informants with whom we spoke suggested that the nature and level of engagement with VSOs was often dependent on the personality of the senior government official responsible for that area (Interview #6: September 8, 2010; Interview #30: February 17, 2011).

Third, while relationships with the voluntary sector are no doubt valued, as evidenced by the prevalence of such relationships in the sector, there is a lack of a mechanism to nurture relationships with the voluntary sector, and to conduct a systematic and transparent review of these relationships to determine their level of effectiveness and satisfaction from the perspectives of the parties involved and to learn from these experiences. Health Canada did conduct a survey on "stakeholder discussions" in 2010, but this was not made public and was carried out as a "one-off" initiative (Interview #30: February 17, 2010). PHAC commissioned a study in 2007 to "identify linkages and gaps in current research on voluntary organizations and volunteers as they relate to health…," and to provide options on how to proceed to fill those gaps, but there does not appear to have been follow-up to this study (Brock et al. 2007).

Fourth, the relationships are typically characterized by a distinct power imbalance between the government agencies and the VSOs. The adversarial and complementary models are not such as to allow for joint planning or inclusive policy-making discussions, and thus tend to keep VSOs on the margins of the development of public policy. Furthermore, as discussed in chapter 3, VSOs are not included in the Pan-Canadian Public Health Network, the central piece of network infrastructure at the national level, to discuss broader public health policy issues (McMillan and Nagpal 2007: 64).

We seem, then, to be some distance away from a clear direction toward what Phillips described as governance by relationship-building. Although partnerships are frequently referenced by the government agencies as being central to public health (see for example, Public Health Agency of Canada 2008: 8), the reality seems to fall far short of this vision. This is not to be unduly critical of PHAC or Health Canada. As discussed earlier in this chapter, there are distinct challenges surrounding the relationships between the voluntary sector and the federal government as a whole. Indeed, the public health sector may well have gone further than most other federal government departments and agencies in reaching out to outside parties.[26] Furthermore, as Hall et al. reported in their survey (2005), the number of VSOs involved in health is particularly high compared to other policy areas in Canada, making the challenge of how to build effective relationships with such a large number rather daunting. Yet, it is clear that much more remains to be done before a model of governance by relationship-building can be realized.

Network governance assumes a much deeper sense of involvement of relevant stakeholders, including the VSOs, than what has been observed in the public health sector to-date at the national level. New mechanisms and behaviours are necessary that are not based primarily on institutional or contractual arrangements, legislation and inflexible forms of accountability (Kamensky et al. 2004: 19). This will not be easy. Without those steps, however, the opportunities for realizing appropriate forms of network governance in the public health area will be lost.

[26] Still, some sectors have developed more elaborate forms of collaboration. Following a review of the roles of NGOs in intergovernmental relations, Julie Simmons identifies the Canadian Council of Ministers of the Environment (CCME) as "the most transparent and systematic of intergovernmental forums in routinely integrating non-governmental actors into its policy development" (Simmons 2008: 367).

CHAPTER 7

GLOBAL DRIVERS

Introduction

U
p to this point, the focus of the book has been on public health governance within Canada. It is, however, important to situate Canada in the global context. It is often pointed out that health issues are not contained within national boundaries. Infectious diseases can start in one remote corner of the world and spread across the planet in a matter of days, sometimes less. Even risk factors linked to chronic diseases, such as cardiovascular disease, cancer and diabetes, are often best understood from a global perspective. In the same way, the Canadian environment is deeply impacted by global trends related to governance issues. It would be an exaggeration to describe trends in global health governance as a form of network governance on a broader scale. Still, the adoption of a more inclusive and collaborative style of governance on the global scene puts pressure on Canada, and other countries, to do likewise by mobilizing and empowering a broader range of actors to participate in public health issues. For non-state actors, in particular, a role on the global stage increases expectations, and possibly opportunities, for involvement at the domestic level.

In this chapter, we will review the emergence of global health governance (GHG), as distinct from international health governance (IHG), present three specific cases which illustrate this shift, and discuss the implications of these developments for public health governance in Canada. As will be discussed, the shift from IHG to GHG is of major significance as it reflects a changing role for the state as it relates to health policy; this is due to the inclusion of a new array of non-state actors, an enhanced role for the World Health Organization (WHO), and the development of more inclusive and, therefore, more complex processes. Through its participation in global health initiatives, Canada can both contribute to and learn from global efforts to address complex governance issues on a broad scale.

Westphalia and beyond

Many scholars trace the basis for international relations, until very recently, back to the Peace of Westphalia of 1648 (Fidler 2004a: 21). Essentially the Peace was articulated a world in which independent sovereign states interact "in a condition of anarchy" (Ibid.: 22). In this case, anarchy does not necessarily mean chaos or disorder, although this can often be the case. Rather, it is meant to convey that the states "do not share or recognize a common, supreme authority" (Ibid.: 22). Although the Peace was intended to end the Thirty Years' War, it succeeded in establishing a framework for international relations that lasted over 300 years. International law, as we know it, "is a Westphalian governance process through which the states create, and consent to be bound by, certain rules of behaviour in connection with their anarchical interactions" (Ibid.: 24). The Westphalian system of international law, then, rests on the principles of sovereignty, non-intervention, and consent (Ibid.: 25).

This is not the place to enter into a detailed treatment of international relations. Broadly speaking, however, the practical consequence of the Westphalian system has been to establish state-centrism as the model for international relations for three centuries. In the establishment of supra-national institutions, such as the United Nations and its related agencies, care was taken to respect the sovereignty of states, and to reflect that these institutions were being established on the basis of the consent of the member states. The Charter of the United Nations (Article 2.1) states clearly that: "The Organization is based on the principle of the sovereign equality of all its members." Furthermore, Article 2.7 states that: "Nothing contained in the present Charter shall authorize the United Nations to intervene in matters which are essentially within the domestic jurisdiction of a state...." "Equality," as applied to the community of nations, of course, is true only in a narrow juridical sense, as opposed to the more relevant 'realpolitik' sense, but for our purposes, what is significant is the expression of the Westphalian model for international relations.

There is nonetheless a strong sense in the literature on international relations that there has been a significant shift over the past half-century (Commission on Global Governance 2005). While the period from the 1940s to the 1970s was characterized by strong reliance on medical science and the lead roles in health policy were taken predominantly by medical elites, by the late 1960s, the "medical model" was being increasingly challenged (Walt and Gilson 1994: 356). New and stronger players came on the global scene that expressed dissatisfaction with the role the states had been playing in international health matters, which expected to have a more direct participation in health policy than was possible previously (Ibid.: 355). Among others, the role of civil society organizations increased both in quantitative and in qualitative terms (Benner et al. 2003).

In terms of sheer numbers, Rosenau refers to an "organizational explosion" which is of no less consequence than the population explosion the world has seen (Rosenau 2005: 47). Using similar terms, Salamon says "a veritable 'association revolution' now seems underway at the global level that may constitute as significant a social and political development of the latter 20th century as the rise of the nation-state was of the latter 19th" (Salamon 1995: 243.). As of 2003, it is estimated that there were 40,000 NGOs operating across borders (Benner et al. 2003: 18). Benner, Reinicke and Witte point to the Johannesburg World Summit on Sustainable Development as reflecting "an ongoing transition to a broader notion of networked governance involving not only governments and international organizations but also businesses and nongovernmental organizations" (Ibid.:18). Indeed, the "roster" of civil society organizations involved in international affairs is impressive and includes international NGOs (INGOs), business-initiated NGOs (BINGOs), little NGOs (LINGOs), and labour-organized NGOs (LONGOs) (Orbinski 2007: 35). Faith-based organizations can also play a major role, such as when the issue of reproductive rights comes to the fore or to help in humanitarian campaigns.

Beyond simply the fact that the non-state participants in international affairs are more numerous, several observers have noted that the processes in which they are involved have changed significantly. In the area of health policy, for example, Lee and Goodman have pointed out that the role of non-state actors, "goes beyond efforts directed at the formal processes of government decision making, in some cases becoming part of the decision-making structure formerly reserved for state actors" (Lee and Goodman 2002: 98). As will be noted below, these developments have seen the emergence of a complex array of global policy networks which may involve, in various combinations, states, NGOs, research organizations, private sector organizations and others, and which have come to play an increasingly important role in the development of health policy at the global level. Moreover, supranational organizations, in particular the World Health Organization (WHO), has seen its role transformed from an agent of member states to an organization which works directly with a wide number of stakeholders, and which is capable of being more assertive in its own right. In response, there have been calls for the development of mechanisms which will regularize these processes, and provide a higher level of accountability and transparency.

From international health governance (IHG) to global health governance (GHG)

As with many other sectors, and perhaps more so than most, the governance of public health on the global stage has undergone a significant transformation over the past few decades. It has gone from the domain of formal relations between states and formal international organizations, primarily the WHO and its regional entities, to one where many more actors take part. Lee et al. refer to a "reterritorialisation" by which "global civil society, virtual communities and cyberspace increasingly defy the logic of territorially defined geography" thus leading to an entirely new set of dynamics (Lee et al. 2002: 6). As Fidler points out: "Global governance incorporates non-state actors and radically differs from state-centric horizontal strategies because it posits that governments alone cannot handle global microbial threats"(Fidler 2004b: 800)

However, the issue is not only relevant in the context of microbial threats, but has a much more general application in public health. Many of the risk factors for chronic diseases such as unhealthy eating, physical activity and obesity, which bedevil many states, particularly the high and middle income countries, and are a reflection of modern society, rather than of conditions present within the borders of any one particular country. As such, strategies to deal with these issues must often cross state boundaries.

It is difficult to pinpoint exactly when the shift from IHG to GHG began in earnest. However, there have been indications from at least the mid-1970s that a progression was taking place. The WHO's initiative of Health for All, as reflected in *Declaration of Alma Alta* of 1978, represents a significant departure from the Westphalian model in that the focus was directly on the welfare of the individual, rather than through the intermediary of the state (Fidler 2004a: 39). In a similar way, the WHO's focus on human rights in relation to the HIV/AIDS pandemic led to a greater role for non-state participants, in particular INGOs, thereby increasing pressure for new governance models globally (Ibid.: 40).

In itself, the participation of INGOs in the WHO is not new. They had been allowed to participate for some time in a category called "official relations." However, this was a limited form of participation, with state actors still having the predominant roles. Increasingly, however, INGOs began to speak outside the formal constraints of the WHO process, as in the case of the International Baby Food Action Network and *Médecins sans frontières*. By 2002, those INGOs participating unofficially were more numerous than those participating through "official relations" (Ibid.: 52-3).

Another factor in the shift from IHG to GHG is in the enhanced role of the WHO to become a factor in the internal affairs of member states. Fidler refers to this as a shift from strictly horizontal (relationship between state actors) to vertical global governance (Ibid.: 37). This is not to suggest that the WHO can dictate how a state responds to certain public health issues. But it does mean that the WHO becomes more centrally involved in how states deal with public health issues. The member state retains its ability to dismiss the advice offered by the WHO, but there can be significant costs for doing so, as will be discussed below in the context of the SARS crisis. The end result is a multi-layered governance regime, which operates both horizontally and vertically, and in which a number of state and non-state actors, either as separate actors or as members of networks, or both, participate with the WHO and other supra-national organizations.

To illustrate the transition from IHG to GHG, we have selected three 21st century cases: the SARS crisis of 2003; the Framework

Convention on Tobacco Control (FCTC) of 2003; and the Global Strategy of Diet, Physical Activity and Health (GS) of 2004. In particular, we will discuss the much more prominent place of non-state actors in public health governance, and the more complex processes to arrive at policy directions due to the presence of non-state actors, as well as the enlarged role of the WHO.[27]

The SARS case was selected because it represents a prominent infectious disease event on a global level, arguably more intense than the more recent (2009) H1N1 pandemic, although the latter caused a greater number of fatalities. The FCTC, and more particularly the process leading up to it, is significant for our purposes because it is the first (and only) public health treaty, and therefore constitutes a so-far unique mechanism to advance public health. The GS is an example of a major initiative to deal with risk factors related to non-infectious, that is, chronic diseases. In different ways, each was a "game-changer" in global public health governance, and therefore worthy of our attention.

The global dimension of SARS

A brief background to the SARS events was provided in chapter 4, so there is no need to repeat it here. From a governance perspective, the SARS crisis is particularly significant because it reflected a fundamental turn in the role of non-state actors in the fight against infectious diseases (Fidler 2004b: 801). Two key elements framed the SARS crisis. First, SARS was a global disease, eventually affecting over 25 countries, and reaching every continent except South America and Antarctica. It quickly jumped over national boundaries, greatly assisted by global airline travel. The second factor was that SARS from the outset was a frightening new disease. It was an atypical virus that the medical community had not seen previously and did not understand how to prevent, treat or contain it (Interview #44: July 7, 2010; Interview #35: October 26, 2010). There was, therefore, a high level of urgency to solve the riddle before it spread further and put the lives of many more people at risk. According to Fidler, SARS "posed a public health governance challenge the likes of which modern public health

---

[27] For this, we draw on the framework for health policy development proposed by Walt and Gilson (1994). This framework, which can also be applied to policy making in other fields, identifies four elements for policy development: actors, processes, context and content. Although all four are critical, we will focus primarily on the first two elements, that is, on actors and processes.

had not previously confronted" (Fidler 2004a: 6). Although in the end, the number of mortalities associated with SARS was not high, relatively speaking, this could not have been known at the beginning. At that point, the focus was on the damage that the virus potentially could inflict.

To this was compounded the fact that in the decades preceding the SARS crisis, public health infrastructure in Canada, as in the United States and in many other countries, had been allowed to weaken. In the US, the influential Institute of Medicine published a report on the subject with the revealing title, *The Disarray of Public Health* (Tilson and Berkowitz 2006: 900). The state of affairs in Canada was no better (McMillan and Nagpal 2007; Lozon and Alikhan 2007; Mowat and Butler-Jones 2007). In Ontario, both the *Campbell* and the *Walker* reports on the SARS crisis documented in graphic detail the sad state of the public health system in that province. Campbell refers to "a broken system," and identifies, among a long list of serious problems, a lack of provincial public health leadership; a lack of laboratory capacity; poor links between the province and hospitals, physicians and nurses; a confused legal framework, the lack of a provincial epidemiological expertise, among other issues (*Campbell Report* 2005a). For Canada, at least, as well as for many other countries which were affected by it, the SARS crisis served as an unfortunate (in the short-term) but effective "wake-up call" (McMillan and Nagpal 2007: 63; Lozon and Alikhan 2007: 53).

How the SARS crisis was handled also had significant reverberations from a global health governance perspective. Seen in this way, SARS' greatest impact was admitting non-state actors as direct participants in the surveillance aspect. The foundation for this had been laid some years previous. In 1997, the World Health Organization agreed to accept infectious disease surveillance reports from non-state sources and, in particular, from the Global Alert Outbreak and Response Network (GOARN). The World Health Assembly, the governing body for the WHO, confirmed this approach in 2001 and re-affirmed it again in 2003, in the midst of the SARS crisis. The ability of the WHO to use data from non-state sources was further reflected in the International Health Regulations which were revised in 2005, and became binding in international law in 2007 (Wilson et al. 2008: 44-45).

GOARN is an epistemic network of over 120 state and non-state actors, established for the purpose of conducting surveillance on infectious disease threats. Participating organizations include research institutions from member states, networks of laboratories, international humanitarian NGOs, Red Cross and Red Crescent societies and others. The acceptance of data from non-state actors was a major step for the WHO, which, consistent with the Westphalian model, previously accepted data only from member states (Fidler 2004a: 133; Interview #44: July 7, 2010). During the SARS events, 152 experts from institutions in 17 countries were providing real-time information on the progression of the virus (David Heymann in Foreword, Ibid.: xiii). According to David Heymann, former Executive Director of Communicable Diseases at the WHO, GOARN proved to be "a catalyst for the successful containment of SARS." (Ibid.: xiv)

The main impetus for the use of GOARN, and consequently of non-state data, during the SARS events was the situation in China. The WHO had strong reason to believe that the Chinese government was not reporting accurately the number of active cases of SARS in that country. Combined with the fact that China was the country most affected by SARS, this risked jeopardizing attempts to understand the virus better and to control it. As Dr. Heymann pointed out, the use of GOARN proved to be highly instrumental in halting the spread of the disease. From a longer-term perspective, the WHO's decision to use surveillance data from non-states, thereby breaking the stranglehold of members states on the control of surveillance data, set a huge precedent and constituted a major step from IHG to GHG.

The second aspect of the SARS crisis that signalled an important change in the governance regime was the use of travel advisories by the WHO. This came about in steps. On March 12, the WHO issued a global alert to raise awareness about cases of unusual respiratory illnesses (Fidler 2004a: 78). This was followed up on March 15 with the issuance of an emergency travel advisory, which reflected an increased concern about a strange new illness, but made no recommendations about restricting travel to any particular locations. It did, however, begin daily postings on the number of reported cases around the world. On April 3, as concern about the disease grew, the WHO issued a travel advisory recommending against non-essential travel to Hong Kong and the Guangdong province of China, because of an infectious disease threat. Never before in its history had the WHO advised against travel to specific geographic regions (Ibid.: 90).

The April 3 travel advisory was followed by a travel advisory on April 23, extending the recommendations against non-essential travel to Beijing and Shanxi province in China and Toronto. What is particularly noteworthy is that this action was done outside the formal role and mandate of the WHO. Furthermore, the WHO took these steps without the approval of the WHA, which only approved the actions of the WHO *ex post facto* (Ibid.: 142). What it meant was that the WHO was taking it upon itself to appeal directly to populations around the world. Member states were neither consulted nor even advised before the travel advisories were issued. In some cases, this led to significant tensions between the WHO and particular countries that were included in the travel advisories. Canada, for one, was quite incensed and publicly objected to being targeted. Ontario, the jurisdiction most affected in Canada by SARS, was particularly vociferous in its objections and the Minister of Health at the time travelled to Geneva to express his concerns in person. These actions may have had an effect in leading the WHO to lift its travel advisories against Canada six days later. Interestingly, those countries which were targeted in WHO's travel advisories, such as Canada and China, questioned the data on which the WHO had based its advisories, but did not question the authority or mandate of the WHO in making them (Ibid.: 142-3). The lack of objection from these countries essentially legitimized the WHO's actions. The act of effectively bypassing member states and speaking directly to populations around the world reflected a new role that the WHO had defined for itself. Many of these new powers were codified in the revised International Health Regulations that were approved in 2005 (Wilson 2008: 44-45).

In the end, the NGOs which became directly involved in the SARS events for the purpose of providing epidemiological data were not numerous, and were quite specialized. Since SARS turned out to be mostly a hospital-based virus, and did not reach the broader community to a significant extent, there was no need for a broader segment of civil society to become involved. Nonetheless, these events constituted an important precedent and signalled a bold new direction for the WHO, with implications for member states and for newly-empowered non-state actors. As Fidler points out:

> *SARS represents the first infectious disease to emerge into a radically new and different global political environment for*

public health...SARS outbreak confirms a transition from old
to new forms of public health governance and teaches lessons
about this transition that are both exciting and sobering
(Fidler 2004a: 7).

In terms of the impact these global developments have
had domestically, it is difficult to make categorical judgments.
Again, because SARS did not involve a huge number of NGOs,
the impact on this level is probably fairly muted. Two points can
nevertheless still be made. First, seeing the WHO accept data from
non-state sources within China seemed to motivate the Chinese
government to reverse itself and begin to report accurately
the progression of the virus within China (Ibid.: 117). It seems
reasonable to conclude that the threat of being circumvented by
other actors pressured the Chinese government into becoming
more transparent and playing a more collaborative role on
the world stage. Second, the threat of the imposition of travel
advisories, and the negative consequences these can have on a
country's economy, provides a strong incentive for member states
to work closely with the WHO to contain infectious diseases that
have the potential to spread globally. Rather than seeing these
diseases as 'national' or local problems, states are now more
likely to see them in a global context and to find strategies to
contain them that involve the WHO and others that form part of
the global community.

Framework Convention on Tobacco Control

The Framework Convention on Tobacco Control (FCTC) represents
the first, and so far the only, WHO-led international treaty in the
area of public health. Interestingly, the treaty was adopted by
the World Health Assembly in May 2003, at about the time that
the SARS crisis was at its peak, and also reflected an important
break from the past. As in the case of SARS, the FCTC was notable
in the extent to which it allowed and, in fact, encouraged, non-
state actors to participate in the process. However, unlike SARS,
the FCTC led to quite a polarized debate, with most states and
NGOs on one side, and large tobacco companies and tobacco
producers, on the other. Moreover, tobacco control involves
a much broader base of stakeholders than was the case with
SARS, and the WHO had a much bigger challenge to construct
the appropriate platforms to accommodate the participation of
all those who had an interest in the issue. Its success in doing

so could well prove to be a turning point for the organization (Taylor 2002). The FCTC represents another clear illustration of the progression from international health governance to global health governance. It also provides an interesting case of how global processes can open fault lines and trigger conflicts that play out at both the global and domestic levels.

Background on the FCTC

Article 19 (2) of the WHO's constitution states that the body has powers to protect and promote international public health, including the power to make treaties (World Health Organization 2009: 2). However, no serious attempt to use the treaty-making powers had been attempted until the 1990s when Dr. Ruth Roemer of the US started on a campaign to use international legal instruments to curb the use of tobacco (Ibid.: 2). The process which followed was a slow one, and followed many stages. Following a number of steps in 1995 and 1996 to build support for the idea, in May 1996, the World Health Assembly (WHA) gave the WHO the mandate to draft a convention (Ibid.: 5). After a period of relative inactivity, the idea was seized by Dr. Gro Harlem Brundtland, then the new Director-General of the WHO, who in 1998 established the Tobacco Free Initiative (TFI) as a special cabinet project. The following year, the WHA established a working group to prepare the draft elements of the treaty. The 2000 meeting of the WHA accepted the provisional texts and called on the intergovernmental negotiating body (INB) to start the negotiations on the convention.

The negotiating process took approximately 2.5 years. During this period, the INB met six times. In between the INB meetings, several consultation sessions were held in many of the WHO regions and sub-regions. On May 21, 2003, the WHA unanimously adopted the FCTC, eight years after the initial resolution to begin the process.

The FCTC contains both demand-side and supply-side provisions. To reduce demand, the convention incorporates:
- protection from exposure to tobacco smoke;
- regulation of the contents of tobacco products;
- regulation of tobacco product disclosures;
- packaging and labelling of tobacco products;
- education, communication, training and public awareness;
- limitations on tobacco advertising, promotion and sponsorship; and

- measures to reduce tobacco dependence and to assist cessation.

To reduce the supply of tobacco, provisions cover:
- illicit trade in tobacco products;
- sales to and by minors; and
- support for economically viable alternative activities (Ibid.: 28).

FCTC through a global governance lens

From a global governance perspective, what is particularly noteworthy about the FCTC is the inclusive process that was followed to lead up to it, which, like SARS, followed a distinctly post-Westphalian path. From the beginning, it was clear that participation in this process would not be restricted to member states. Dr. Ruth Roemer, who proposed the idea, was a law professor and not part of the WHO machinery. Moreover, a number of NGO stakeholders, beginning with the American Public Health Association, were quick to mobilize and saw a role for themselves in the public debate. In response, tobacco companies – the major ones of which are Philip Morris, British American Tobacco and Japan Tobacco International – also mobilized quickly and sought every avenue to derail the treaty process (Collin 2004: 94; Mamudu et al. 2008).

Underscoring the inclusive nature of this process, the WHO conducted public hearings on the convention in 2000. This was the *first time* in WHO's history that such hearings had been held (Collin 2004: 93). One hundred and forty-four organizations testified in these hearings, including tobacco control NGOs as well as tobacco companies and tobacco producers. In addition, 500 written submissions were received. Beyond this, the WHO accelerated the process by which INGOs could enter into 'official relations' with the WHO (Ibid.: 93). To underscore the point, one of the guiding principles (Article 4, no.7) of the FCTC states: "The participation of civil society is essential in achieving the objective of the Convention and its protocols (cited in Mamudu and Glantz 2009: 164).

Perhaps the most significant element to illustrate the post-Westphalian nature of the process is the establishment, by the WHO, of the Framework Convention Alliance (FCA), which Keck and Selkirk have called a "transnational advocacy network framework" (cited in Mamudu and Glantz, Ibid.: 151). Rather than simply advocating for the convention, however, the FCA had a place in the actual development of the instrument and played a major role in influencing the member state actors in the process (Ibid.: 151). The WHO was the catalyst for the creation of the FCA by giving a grant to Action on Smoking and Health, a UK-based NGO, to explore how to involve civil society in the negotiations (Ibid.: 152). What emerged was a loose coalition of NGOs that expanded considerably in the course of the process, going from 72 in 2000 to 306 organizations from 98 countries in 2008 (Ibid.: 153). Although the FCA did not have 'official relation' status with the WHO, it used its observer position to address the formal meetings, make proposals, comment on the proposals of others, in addition to engaging in active lobbying in the corridors. At each INB, the FCA circulated among the delegates side by side analyses of the draft texts, with suggested alternative wording and accompanying rationale. These came to be viewed quite positively and relied upon by many of the delegates to help formulate their positions in the negotiations (Wilkenfeld 2005: 22). In fact, the FCA was so effective as to cause the states opposing the convention, principally the US, to complain about the influence it was having (Mamudu and Glantz 2009: 156). One of its most powerful tactics was the use of the *Alliance Bulletin*, an Internet-based communications product that came out on a daily basis, and which proved to be quite effective in framing the debate around the convention (Ibid.: 154). Although the FCA was effectively excluded from the final INB, it continued to participate indirectly by maintaining its relationships with sympathetic delegations and continuing to provide them with draft texts and rationales (Wilkenfeld 2005: 30).

The FCTC process, then, was quite a radical departure from the state-centric approach of the Westphalian model. It is true that in the end, the process became closed, and only member states were able to vote on whether to approve and, subsequently, to ratify, the convention. However, the processes leading up to those decision points included hundreds of stakeholders who were directly and substantively involved in developing the convention. Moreover, because tobacco control issues, like public health issues generally, touch on many other sectors, the FCTC process broadened the constituency of organizations typically involved in health issues to include actors from other areas, such as economics, law, trade, education and environment (Collin et al. 2005: 261). The process leading up to the FCTC, then, is a clear instance of international health governance transforming itself into global health governance (Ibid.: 263).

A second point to be observed is the impact of the convention on the domestic scene in many countries. The FCTC points to the limitations of national governance on a global issue. Tobacco consumption, as a global issue, needs a global response, which is what the convention tries to provide (Ibid.: 267). At the same time, however, the FCTC process added another layer of complexity within many of the countries that were involved in that it helped to motivate a number of NGOs – examples in Canada include Physicians for a Smoke-Free Canada and the Heart and Stroke Foundation of Canada – to become involved in the issue, and to attempt to influence the positions taken by their respective national governments (Interview #4: June 24, 2010). National-level meetings took place in many countries to help formulate that country's position on the proposed convention. The result was that a global issue became a domestic one (Mamudu and Glantz 2009: 154).

Again, the FCA was a significant contributing factor in this. An important part of the FCA tactics in countering the positions of those states who were opposing the convention was, through their member organizations, to inform the public of their government's positions and help local organizations to lobby those governments to change their stance (Ibid.: 161). In the US, for example, NGOs such as the American Lung Association, the American Cancer Society and the Campaign for Tobacco-Free Kids, among many others, all took a strong interest in the convention, and exerted pressure on the US government to change its anti-convention position or, if it was unwilling to do so, at least to withdraw from the FCTC negotiations so as not to impede the development of the convention (Wilkenfeld 2005: 31). The US government then found itself between deeply opposing interests, with large tobacco companies on one side and a broad constituency of NGOs on the other.[28] The Japanese government was in a similar position, with the Japanese Medical Association and other NGOs strongly pressing the government to reverse its opposition to the convention, and the Japanese Tobacco Inc.,

---

[28] The US eventually voted in favour of approving the convention when it saw that its position had almost no support from other countries. To date, however, it has yet to ratify the convention.

and its supporters pressing in the opposite direction (Mamudu and Glanz 2009: 161).[29] Of course, the implementation phase of the FCTC also impacted the relations at the domestic level as governments around the world have had to introduce or modify tobacco control measures and often to increase regulation on the sale and use of tobacco products (Collin 2004: 95).

In Canada, the domestic and global dimensions of the process leading up to the convention were closely intertwined. In this case, the Canadian government, led by Health Canada, was a leading proponent of the FCTC from the outset. Rather than trying to play a mediating role between the NGO community and the tobacco industry, the government took an active role in building a constituency of support for the initiative. One government informant recounted how, using Canadian NGOs as intermediaries, the Canadian government directed financial support to NGOs in strategically placed countries as a way of encouraging the support of these NGO communities for the convention. The same informant also advised that Health Canada worked closely with Canadian NGOs to gain intelligence from their networks about the positions and strategies of international NGOs on the various issues under negotiation (Interview #19: October 12, 2010).

As a global leader in the fight against tobacco consumption, Canada did not experience sharp new divisions as a result of the FCTC. In a large measure, the provisions contained in the convention reflected steps that had already been taken in Canada as a result of decades of tobacco cessation activities. The large multinational cigarette companies preferred to target countries, often low-income states, they believed would be more sympathetic to their interests or could be influenced to be so (Mamudu et al. 2008: 1696). Still, opposition to the convention did manifest itself in Canada to some extent. The tobacco industry was invited to consultations on the issue held by Health Canada and used the occasions to advocate alternative approaches. Representatives of the tobacco growers also played a fairly active role (Interview #19: October 12, 2010). Finally, the large tobacco companies sought to influence governments indirectly by attempting to shape public opinion, for example by supporting individuals or groups willing to critique *Curbing the Epidemic: Governments and the Economics*

---

[29] This is a particularly tangled situation, as the Japanese Finance Ministry owned about half the firm.

of Tobacco Control (CTE), the World Bank's pivotal study on the economics of tobacco control (Mamudu et al. 2008: 1695).

Global Strategy for Diet, Physical Activity and Health

The third case which signals a recent shift from IHG to GHG is the Global Strategy for Diet, Physical Activity and Health (GS). The GS, which was approved by the World Health Assembly in May 2004, was initiated as a result of concern about the increase in the incidence of non-communicable disease, or chronic diseases, particularly in low-income countries. A resolution on the issue was first passed in 2000. The 2002 World Health Report reinforced concern around the issue by revealing common risk factors of many chronic diseases, such as cancer, cardio-vascular disease, diabetes and many others. The common risk factors identified – unhealthy eating, physical inactivity and tobacco use – showed that many of these diseases were preventable (Norum 2005: 83). In that year, it was decided to develop a global strategy to lower the incidence of chronic disease and to submit this to the World Health Assembly meeting in 2004. At its core, therefore, the GS was a chronic disease prevention strategy.

The GS process

The GS did not attract the same level of attention, in Canada or abroad, as the FCTC.[30] Unlike the FCTC, it is not a treaty or formal convention, so it had no status in international law. Consequently, there were no enforcement mechanisms; it was meant to persuade, not compel, the actions of member states. Nevertheless, the process leading to the GS resembles in many respects that for the FCTC. In both cases, there was a battle between public health advocates and the corporate sector, albeit with a lower level of intensity than in the case of the FCTC. As with the FCTC, the debate around the GS was not confined to the international sector with a supranational agency, in this case, the WHO, attempting to find a consensus. In fact, it was played out on a much broader canvas. The WHO document detailing the process followed for the GS reveals a commitment to a broad level of stakeholder involvement from the outset. In this vein, there were four tracts to the consultation phase: consultations with member states, which were carried out by the

---

[30] Comparing the dimensions of the two, one key informant referred to the FCTC as the "pumpkin," whereas the GS was the "orange" (Interview #19: October 12, 2010).

six WHO regions; consultations with UN agencies, including the FAO, the World Bank, the World Trade Organization and many others; consultations with civil society organizations, including not-for-profit organizations and professional organizations in the area of health, physical activity and nutrition; and consultations with the private sector, including the food, non-alcoholic beverage, sport and advertising industries.

In reality, the process was far from being a level playing field. The food industry, particularly the sugar industry and the manufacturers of confectionary goods and beverages, organized strong lobbies to pressure supranational organizations such as the WHO, the WTO and the FAO, as well as the governments of many states where these industries had a strong presence, in particular the US. On the other hand, NGOs concerned about public health had a much more difficult time getting their voices heard. One observer, frustrated with the influence the corporate sector was able to exert, complained that the NGOs were being treated "not so much as partners as peons" (Cannon 2004: 377).

Nevertheless, what is significant for our purposes is the WHO's recognition that in order for the GS to be effective and legitimate, it (the WHO) needed to reach beyond member states. Writing on behalf of the WHO, Amalia Waxman says that: "One of the strategy's most important conclusions is that reducing the burden of NCDs requires a multi-sectoral, multi-stakeholder approach" (Waxman 2005: 164). While the responsibility for implementing the GS rests primarily with states (Tukuitonga and Keller 2005: 122), Waxman argues that this is not sufficient "in an increasingly globalized and interdependent world," and that the GS's goals "can only be met through decisive and coherent action by countries, sustained political commitment, and broader, multi-level involvement with all relevant stakeholders worldwide" (Waxman 2005: 166).

The WHO's advocacy role in the GS

What is also particularly noteworthy is the role the WHO gave itself in this process. The organization saw itself as far more than a facilitator, mediator, or catalyst for member states. Rather it positioned itself explicitly as an advocate in the quest for improved public health and a leader in the process of achieving better health outcomes. In this context, the WHO process document deserves to be quoted at length:

Countries and their peoples must be alerted to the health problems caused by unhealthy diets and physical inactivity, of the devastating social and economic outcomes of chronic conditions resulting from these risk factors and to the proven prevention interventions. The involvement of different stakeholders will allow an opportunity to ensure that this information is adequately provided to decision-makers, the public, and above all, the participants of the process. Communication of this information, therefore, will be an essential facet in the process leading to a strategy document. **WHO will address this need to inform, convince and mobilize stakeholders continuously in the course of the development of the Strategy**" (World Health Organization 2003a: 2 – emphasis added).

This role as an advocate for public health, therefore, compels the WHO to reach beyond the member states to engage a broader public so that the needed reforms can be achieved and successfully implemented. The WHO's self-defined role to "convince and mobilize stakeholders" is clearly far beyond a Westphalian concept of international relations.

The debate over the GS also had reverberations at the national state level. As mentioned earlier, there is clear evidence of a strong lobbying campaign by parts of the corporate sector on member states. The argument advanced was that governments should not be intruding on the personal lifestyle choices of their citizens. Fears were also raised about the damage that could be caused to the economies particularly of sugar producing countries. In the US, the Sugar Association and the confectionery industry wrote to US Secretary of Health, Tommy Thompson, to demand that the US withdraw its financial support to the WHO if that organization persisted with the GS (Norum 2005: 85). Similar letters were sent by the Corn Refiners' Association, International Dairy Foods Association, National Corn Growers' Association, Snack Food Association, Sugar Association, Wheat Foods Council and US Council of International Business. In response to these pressures, the office of the US Secretary of Health wrote to the WHO to seek to stall the development of the GS (Ibid.: 85)

Industry organizations were also active among the G77, a loose coalition of low and middle income countries, essentially advancing the argument that the GS would damage the economic development of many of those countries (Ibid.: 85). The fact that arguments made by these organizations were taken up by the G77 countries and articulated at the WHO Executive Board meeting in January 2004 and to the FAO Committee of Agriculture meeting in February of that year is evidence of the influence the industry associations exerted on these countries.

While these actions were taking place, the public health organizations in the US were working hard in support of making the GS as strong as possible. The American Cancer Society, for example, wrote to Dr. Lee Jong-Wook, Director General of the WHO, to express their support for the strategy. Furthermore, a group of US senators took it upon themselves to write to Tommy Thompson to express their support for the GS and the principles it reflected (Margetts 2004: 362).

As mentioned, the debate in Canada around the GS was not as divisive as was the case in the US. The stakes were clearly not as high as was the case with the FCTC. Partially for that reason, and because their resources were limited, major public health NGOs, such as the Canadian Cancer Society and the Heart and Stroke Foundation, focussed most of their energies on the FCTC (Interview #6: September 8, 2010). Some professional associations, such as the Dieticians of Canada, took a more active interest in the GS, as well as the Canadian chapter of the Centre for Science in the Public Interest (Interview #9: September 22, 2010; Interview #53: June 24, 2011). On the other side, industry representatives, such as the Sugar Institute of Canada, pressed their cases in the opposite direction with a view to either stopping the provisions of the GS or at least weakening its wording (Interview #9: September 22, 2010). Although the debate was not as intense in Canada as in some other countries, particularly the US, it did accentuate pre-existing fault lines in Canada and contributed to an already complex policy environment at the domestic level.

The drive for collaborative mechanisms

From the global governance perspective, the three case studies suggest that the number and the range of participants that are involved in global health policy processes have increased dramatically. Furthermore, in each of the cases reviewed, processes related to public health at the global level were no longer restricted to nation states, with supranational institutions such as the WHO playing a coordinating role. In the cases of the GS and the FCTC, direct and strategic involvement from NGOs and the corporate sector was clearly in evidence. This was somewhat less the case with the SARS crisis, because, as discussed, it was not an issue which lent itself to broad societal involvement. Even here, however, the involvement of non-state parties in the collection of vital surveillance data constituted a fundamental break from the past. What's more, in its use of travel advisories, the WHO went over the heads of member states to speak directly to the travelling public, thus signalling a new role for itself.

In both the FCTC and GS cases, the WHO dealt directly and intensively with INGOs and BINGOs. The involvement of these parties went beyond simple consultation. Rather, they were substantively involved in the development of the instruments in question. Overall, these cases saw the emergence of governance mechanisms and processes that are more suited to a broader and more diverse community of participants – in other words, that reflect the transition to more collaborative forms of governance. This reflects, as Slaughter has observed about global processes more generally, that "public and private actors are coming together to develop new ways of decision-making under conditions of complexity" (Slaughter 2004: 194).

Does this mean that the scope for nations has been reduced? The changes in technology and communications that accompanied globalization have led to what one observer has called "rampant fragmentation of norms, ideologies, values, and institutions" (Kettl 2000: 491). Kettl points out that "National sovereignty has shrunk along with government's capacity to understand and shape the emerging issues and the conflicts that underlie them" (Ibid.: 492). In a similar vein, Dodgson, Lee and Drager have referred to the "decapitating of the state" (Dodgson et al. 2002: 8).

Yet care must be taken to avoid overstating the case. The role of states in global processes remains critical. Member states continue to be the voting members at the World Health Assembly (Constitution of the World Health Organization, chapter III). Similarly, the ratification of treaties, as was discussed in relation to the Framework Convention on Tobacco Control, can only be carried out by member states.

It is more accurate to say that the role of national governments has become more complicated at the global level. The proliferation of organizations active in global issues, and the networks that have been formed among many of these participants, has meant that states, while remaining "primary agents" (Weiss 2005: 73), have had to find space for other parties in the various decision-making processes. States have had to work with and within networks to address complex issues, at times in leadership roles, in others as participants with many others. Rather than replacing governments, networks involving states, representatives of civil society, epistemic communities and industry groups, among others, have become a supplement to state governments as well as to the formally established international organizations, such as the UN and the WHO (Reinicke 1999-2000: 51; Benner et al. 2003: 21; Scholte 2002: 337).

Reflecting on changes in the global international scene, former U.N. Secretary-General Kofi Annan said in 2006:

> I believe these global policy networks, capable of bringing together Governments, civil society and the private sector, are the most promising partnerships of our globalizing age. They work for inclusion and reject hierarchy. They help set agendas and frame debates. They develop understanding and disseminate knowledge (Annan 2006).

Global networks provide an enormous opportunity to bridge policy differences and to achieve outcomes that reflect the interests and concerns of a broader cross-section of stakeholders. Used well, they can harness "the positive power of conflict"[31] (Slaughter 2004: 195). Reinicke and Deng speak to the potential of global policy networks in saying that "using them [global networks] wisely will no doubt improve our ability to cope with the difficult challenges posed by rapid global liberalization, technological change, and the complexity these trends have brought to our lives" (Reinicke and Deng 2000: 5). Networks are well positioned "to take maximum advantage of the tensions and differences among disparate groups"(Reinicke 1999-2000: 55). Ultimately, global networks are a part of the new reality that has transformed the global scene in public health, as well as in many other policy sectors.

Along similar lines, Boutris Boutris-Ghali, Annan's predecessor, stated: "The time of absolute and exclusive sovereignty have passed" (cited in Weiss 2005: 69). The question that now presents itself is what has replaced "absolute and exclusive sovereignty," particularly as it relates to public health. Unfortunately, there does not appear to be a pre-established road-map to follow. From all appearances, the new processes and

---

[31] To balance the picture, there also exists 'dark networks,' which are dedicated to illegal activities, such as drug or people trafficking and terrorism.

mechanisms are *ad hoc* constructions, suited to the exigencies of the particular case in question. In many ways, global public health actors are having to re-invent the rules of the game while it is in play. Networks are being formed, but there is not yet a consistent pattern of network-building; rather, these develop differently according to different circumstances and conditions and with different combinations of actors (Reinicke and Deng 2000: 4-5; Kahler 2009). In the same 2006 speech cited earlier, Kofi Annan said: "The United Nations' involvement with [...] networks has been extensive. We must now move forward, from largely unplanned interaction towards a more systematic approach – while maintaining the flexibility that is one of civil society's greatest assets."

The challenge Annan presents is not a trivial one. Global networks are not a panacea. As discussed in chapter 2, networks come with a significant level of risk. Benner et al. include in the risks that pertain to the global context such factors as: large numbers of participants raising questions about manageability and transaction costs; the possibility of creating or accentuating existing unequal access and power, particularly affecting low income countries; encouraging "lowest common denominator" solutions as a function of the need for compromise; and polarized views that cannot be reconciled, leading to paralysis (Benner et al. 2003: 21). Perhaps more fundamental still are questions related to transparency, legitimacy, equity, fairness, accountability and evaluation. Success in addressing these challenges is contingent on what Witte et al. have called "the effective application of a minimum set of rules" (Witte et al. 2003: 15), which have yet to be developed.

Moreover, several authors have pointed to the need for actors to hone specific skill sets for the new mechanisms of global governance to succeed (Kickbusch et al. 2007: 230; Benner et al. 2003; Slaughter 2004). Since "hard power" of international legal instruments has now has been at least partially displaced by "soft power" of guidelines, best practices and principles, which are more typical of policy networks (Slaughter 2004: 178), participants need to become more skilled at "leading from behind" (Reinicke 1999-2000: 54), that is, influencing rather than commanding.

What some authors have called the current state of "laissez-faire" (Witte et al. 14) needs to be improved. More appropriate, yet rigorous accountability measures and useful evaluations need to be developed and applied. Weiss is quite right in suggesting that we need to think about ways "to pool the collective strengths and avoid the collective weaknesses of governments, intergovernmental organizations, NGOs and global civil society" (Weiss 2005: 83). The question remains, how to do this most effectively? Certainly there will be many concrete achievements as well as false starts. As Rosenau suggests: "All one can conclude with confidence is that in the twenty-first century the paths to governance will lead in many directions, some that will emerge into sunlit clearings and others that will descend into dense jungles" (Rosenau 1995: 64).

Conclusion: Implications for Canada

From a Canadian health governance perspective, many of the above-mentioned key challenges associated with GHG parallel those that confront network governance at the domestic level. In both cases, the central question is how to achieve a more pluralist yet cohesive system of governance (Dodgson et al. 2002: 23). Just as there needs to be a framework to include state and non-state actors in global health matters, the same applies to the Canadian scene. Both contexts, for example, call for a pluralistic approach to accountability, although the application of that concept may need to be adjusted to suit the circumstances.

To return to the point raised in the opening paragraph of this chapter, the line between public health governance at the global and domestic levels is both blurred and porous. This is not to deny the importance of context as an important element in policy making, as reflected in the framework proposed by Walt and Gilson. The range of actors and circumstances of the global scene, as well as the vast scale, make the challenges related to the global scene that much greater. Still, the knowledge acquired and skills developed through working in partnership with non-state actors, and in participating in complex, multi-layered processes, are transferable between the global and the domestic fronts and, indeed, are mutually reinforcing. As an active participant in public health governance processes, both domestically and globally, Canada is in a good position both to share the knowledge it has acquired, and to learn from the experiences of others about effective practices and mechanisms.

To take the analysis a step further, it is not a great inferential leap to argue that Canada's participation in GHG, including its role in the FCTC and the GS, tends to fuel the drive for collaborative mechanisms in Canada. National governments must now contend with a broader number of players, in particular from civil society, who has the sophistication, knowledge and the opportunity to participate in global processes and to bring these battles back to the domestic stage. An organization which becomes involved in a global process will often see itself as a "player" on the domestic scene as well and will tend to intervene with the domestic government with a greater level of confidence and legitimacy. Moreover, a national government dismisses these players at its own risk. The FCTC and the GS provide examples of NGOs, in this case mostly in the US, strategizing with foreign governments and INGOs against the positions taken by their own governments because they could not get what they considered to be a sympathetic hearing from that government (Collin 2004; Cannon 2004; Norum 2005; Wilkenfeld 2005). Even when the relationships are more positive, such as that between Health Canada and the NGOs it funded to allow them to participate in the FCTC process, the NGOs felt empowered at times to publicly criticize the government and to take positions which were, from Health Canada's perspective, extreme and unhelpful (Lencucha et al. 2010: 79; Interview #19: October 12, 2010). As stated earlier, there is probably no going back to the ways of Westphalian public health (Witte et al. 2003: 185). It can be expected that participation in global policy initiatives will fuel the expectations from NGOs and industry groups that they will be players in policy process. How Canada chooses to respond in the short-term remains to be seen. However, it seems likely that, over time, these circumstances will put pressure on Canada to develop further its collaborative mechanisms, practices and skills for both the domestic and the global environments.

IV – DEVELOPING THE TOOLS

CHAPTER 8

FACING THE TOUGH QUESTIONS

Introduction

I n previous chapters, we have attempted to identify the governance challenges inherent in public health in Canada, and have argued that a network governance approach might hold the key to successfully addressing these challenges. Yet, a sceptic might question whether network governance is good as a practical concept or just good theory. Can the obstacles to operationalizing this concept be overcome in the 'real' world? This chapter and the next one will focus on the more practical side of network governance and attempt to show that while the obstacles are numerous and considerable, they are not insurmountable.

In this chapter, we examine three objections that can be raised about the practicality of network governance. The first relates to the governability question. In other words, is not some form of overall direction needed to prevent society from descending into chaos and, if this is so, how and by whom would this direction be applied? The second question deals with the related issues of legitimacy, accountability and transparency. Allowing that network governance could be operationalized, our persistent sceptic might ask, how might it not become run by elites who are hidden from view and unaccountable to anyone except perhaps each other? The third question asks how network governance in public health is possible when it is situated within the largely hierarchical structure of the government of Canada? In other words, to borrow terminology from Hubbard and Paquet, can "small g" governance find a place in "Big G" government (Hubbard and Paquet 2010: 1)?

Network governance and the 'governability' question

Implied in network governance is a notion of the changing role of the state. Much has been written about how the role of the modern state is changing, and there is no need to treat this question extensively here. For our purposes, suffice it to say the level of complexity of modern society is such that it is no longer realistic to expect governments to control all the levers to address policy issues on their own, nor is it acceptable to govern as if all power is vested in the public authority. The state must now see itself in a more diverse role, and one that involves closer association with a number of other actors. In some cases, it would mean working as a participant among others in various processes; in other cases, it would take more of a leadership role. Even in the latter instances, however, it must often lead more by influencing, motivating and incentivizing people to act, rather than by relying on its powers to command-and-control. As Stoker put it: "Government needs to learn to steer with a light touch, and the capacity and skills to act in such a way will have to be installed in governance systems" (Stoker 2006: 52). It is in this context that *metagovernance* becomes an important notion to allow network governance to move forward.

Metagovernance has been defined as "a way of enhancing coordinated governance in a fragmented political system based on a high degree of autonomy for a plurality of self-governing networks and institutions." As opposed to a command-and-control approach, it is "an indirect form of governing that is exercised by influencing various processes of self-governance" (Sorensen 2006: 100). A key condition of metagovernance is that the state must give up the notion that it is (or should be) in complete control. What emerges in its place is a stronger notion of shared control. Pierre and Peters rightly point out that "the best proof of the state's leverage and its political capabilities is not whether it can accomplish desired changes in society by itself but whether it is able to muster the resources and forge the coalitions necessary to attain the goals at all" (Pierre and Peters 2000: 197). Ultimately, this reflects a shrinking 'span of control' by the state, which is off-set by an expanding 'span of influence,' as governments are called upon to participate in an increasing number of processes and conversations on public policy questions (O'Toole 2010: 8). Ideally, the end result is a government more attuned to the views and needs of the population, and a more engaged and empowered citizenry.

It follows from this that states need a new tool kit to exercise this form of leadership. In this light, Sorensen and Torfing have proposed four elements of metagovernance (Sorensen and Torfing 2009: 248). The first is "network design," which seeks "to influence the scope, character, composition and institutional procedures of the networks" (Ibid.: 246). This could mean creating new networks or working with those already in existence. In either case, a particularly important role for the state is to ensure the inclusion in the process of all relevant parties, particularly those from more marginalized parts of society. Without this safeguard, networks are vulnerable to the tendency to become social élites, and therefore to speak primarily for those parts of society which are already in the strongest positions. In this context, the role of the state is to ensure a relatively level playing field, so that the more disadvantaged parts of society have an opportunity to make their voices heard, and that the policy options they present are considered seriously.

Second, "network framing" is about influencing the "political goals, fiscal conditions, legal basis and discursive story-line of the networks" (Ibid.: 246). This includes facilitating coordination, as well as monitoring the performance of the network and communicating its effectiveness with network members. In many cases, these functions would fall to the state. In others, the state might use its influence to ensure that these are carried out, without having to take on this role itself.

The third aspect is "network management," which refers "to attempts to reduce tensions, resolve conflicts, empower particular actors and lower the transaction costs in networks" (Ibid.: 247). This could mean ensuring that all participants have a fair chance of engaging in the discussions; finding ways to resolve conflicts; providing resources where necessary; and circulating information about the work of the network to ensure transparency. This is not to cast the role of the state as the 'chief puppeteer' of the process, seeking to control the actions of the other parties through financial or other inducements. To do so would essentially undo the whole purpose of governance through networks and, over time, would discourage rather than encourage authentic dialogue.

Nevertheless, there is a need for some basic machinery for a network approach to function effectively, which, in many cases, the state is in the best position to provide.

Finally, Sorensen and Torfing include "network participation," by which they mean attempting "to influence the policy agenda, the range of options, the premises for decision making and the negotiated policy options" (Ibid.: 247). It is not necessary for the state to come up with the major policy ideas to address the issues under consideration. In many cases, it may be that most of the new and innovative approaches come from other parties, and that the role of the state is to act more as a facilitator, convenor and stage-setter. It can also appropriately position itself as an advocate of open discussion of all alternative options (Ibid.: 246-247). Moreover, this role does not preclude the state from having and expressing its own views. In addition, because the state party is often well-positioned to take into account the major interests and viewpoints surrounding an issue, it can, as Sorensen and Torfing suggest, play an important role in facilitating the process through agenda-setting and the development of options. Put broadly, the role of the state becomes helping to establish the circumstances under which an inclusive, open and informed discussion can take place, and to some extent, to smooth the way towards a policy outcome that will have broad-based support.

Metagovernance, then, provides a style of governance that is more subtle and indirect than what is traditionally seen in "Big G" government. Public authorities, elected and non-elected, need to resist the temptation to steer "governance networks in ways that eliminate their capacity for self-regulation" (Ibid.: 246), and thereby defeat the potential advantage they bring. Admittedly, in some areas, such as law enforcement, border control and defence, the means of governing will need to be more direct. In other areas, it is more a question of mobilizing societal forces regarding public policy issues and facilitating processes to decide how those issues should be resolved.

One might legitimately question the efficiency of this form of governance. There is no doubt, as discussed in chapter 2, that network governance approaches require a greater investment of time at the front end. Public discussion of complex public policy issues are bound to be protracted, fractious and messy. Yet there is no simple way of resolving complex problems. What makes a policy issue 'wicked' is precisely that its level of complexity allows no simple solution. A state may use its authority to impose a solution, but unless it has been the subject of a broad discussion involving the major interests, the chances are high that this 'solution' will be short-lived. On the other hand, using the tools of metagovernance in the context of network governance increases the chances for a more satisfactory and more sustainable solution. As Bogason and Musso put it: "Metagovern or perish!" (Bogason and Musso 2005: 13).

Accountability, transparency and legitimacy

Network governance inevitably raises issues of the closely interrelated issues of accountability, transparency and legitimacy. Until it can be clarified to whom, how and for what, a network is accountable – its accountability, transparency and, hence, its legitimacy will be in question. To begin, accountability is a term which has seen many different interpretations and usages. In one of the clearest definitions, accountability is seen as "the relationship between an actor and a forum, in which the actor has an obligation to explain and justify his or her conduct; the forum can pose questions and pass judgment, and the actor may face consequences" (Bovens et al. 2008: 225). The difficulty is that many of the existing tools for accountability are based on a hierarchical model of government and are ill-suited for the collaborative forms of governance that are arising (Kettl 2002: 499). In its conventional application, accountability asks who is in charge. Under network governance, however, the answer is that "many are somewhat in charge" (Agranoff 2007: 191). The result is that accountability gets "lost in the cracks of horizontal and hybrid governance" that are more typical of modern governance (Bovens et al. 2008: 240).

Using a conventional approach to assess accountability in forms of collaborative governance can mean either imposing unnecessary and counter productive constraints over those governance arrangements, or disconnecting those assessments from a sense of what is actually happening. This could mean losing the potential to evaluate the benefit that network governance can bring, or putting public officials in a position where they are using accountability measures that are at odds with how business is conducted in reality, and in so doing, creating fictitious constructs. To illustrate, in many present day regimes, it is not uncommon for managers to be held 'accountable' for programs and policies over which they have limited control, because of the number of other actors involved (Kettl 2002: 493). On a broader level, Van Kersbergen and Van Waarden ask "whether a minister's formal responsibility for actions already taken by his civil servants (that he did not and could not have known about) are becoming more and more a strange legal fiction as the size and differentiation of the administration increases and as decisions are increasingly taken in networks of actors located at different levels of aggregation in both the public and private spheres" (Van Kersbergen and Van Waarden 2004: 157).

Network governance requires a different approach to accountability. In the first instance, there needs to be recognition that governance has become a "team sport" (Salamon 2002: 600). In many instances, it is no longer possible to ascribe a policy or program intervention to one particular person, or one particular agency. As Pierre and Peters have pointed out, the "problem" of many hands "is endemic in public life" (Pierre and Peters 2005: 131). Rather, the authorship of a product is often the result of the combined activities of a number of different organizations which may be only indirectly linked to each other. What is needed at the outset is a recognition that the defining characteristic of the new tools of governance "is their indirect character, their establishment of interdependencies between public agencies and a host of third-party actors" (Salamon 2002: 11).

Where does this leave the question of accountability? Essentially, it means that we need to change our application of this concept. The type of accountability that reflects a linear, mono-centric type of structure is no longer appropriate. Indeed, as Goldsmith and Eggers have pointed out, traditional accountability measures clash with the very purpose of networks, which is to provide decentralized, flexible, and creative responses to public problems (Goldsmith and Eggers 2004: 123). More pluralistic concepts of accountability are needed which recognize new social and political realities (Salamon 2002: 38). What is emerging is the notion that the relationship between the "accountability holder" and the "accountability holdee" needs to be less distanced and formal, and more interactive than has been the case under the traditional model (Aarsæther et al. 2009: 579). This requires a kind of leadership in which the leader is "organically part of the system rather than outside it" (Stoker 2006: 52). In the context of modern governance, legitimate power means "power with," not "power over," the citizenry (Bogason et al. 2002: 687). In fact, this approach to accountability, which R.C. Box calls "collaborative discourse," becomes the foundation for political legitimacy (Box 2002: 34).

How, then, can these notions be operationalized? Aarsæther and his colleagues helpfully propose three levels of accountability as it relates to networks: "upwards," that is, to the elected representatives, through a combination of hands-on and hands-off mechanisms consistent with metagovernance; "outward," to the affected stakeholders, through the openness of their processes and their ability to generate and share information; and "downwards," to the citizenry at large, by making reports of their activities public, and through a willingness to explain and debate their policy positions openly (Aarsæther et al. 2009: 581-582).

Admittedly, accountability in a network governance context is a more complex undertaking than in more hierarchical applications. New tools are needed to account for the fact that modern governance is often multilevel, indirect, and based on interdependencies between public agencies and several third-party actors (Salamon 2002: 11). The means tools to evaluate the democratic component of networks can be drawn from the three-level classification of network accountability Aarsæther et al. have proposed, such as open discussions with stakeholders and public reporting. Others can be added to these. Kettl stresses the importance of information and "creating new mechanisms to generate, assess, and manage this information" (Kettl 2002: 492).

"Value-for-money" evaluations characteristic of new public management are useful in some contexts, but are limiting and potentially misguided if applied indiscriminately. What become more central are indicators relating to finding and removing disincentives to nonparticipation, reducing interaction costs, promoting transparency, and securing commitment to joint activities (Posner 2002: 546). Network governance requires measures not just for policy outputs, but also for process-related elements, such as fairness, justice, participation, and articulation of shared interests (Denhardt and Denhardt 2002: 133).

What is significant for our purposes is not to settle on a particular set of criteria to evaluate the democratic component of network governance, but rather to argue that it is feasible to set such criteria. This is not to suggest that the more traditional accountability mechanisms are irrelevant. More likely, what is needed in the current circumstances is a blend of old and new forms of accountability. Networks, in and of themselves, do not ensure greater accountability. They can be accountable or not, with many degrees in between. What is important is to ensure that they are accompanied by systems of upward, outward and downward accountability as Aarsæther et al. have suggested. With the appropriate accountability measures in place, enforced by broader participation of stakeholders (Bogason and Musso 2006: 15), networks can contribute to liberal democracy by creating new opportunities for what some have called "authentic public participation" (King et al. 1998: 317).

Accountability in network governance, interwoven as it is with issues of legitimacy and transparency, while complex, is not impossible. Admittedly, much needs to be done before liberal democracies have a clearer sense of how to balance and blend the different accountability systems that can be put in play. Pierre and Peters accurately point out that "we still have not developed a model of political accountability in a governance perspective" (Pierre and Peters 2005: 127). From a practical perspective, applicable to public health and many other circumstances, two major considerations should be kept in mind. First, what should be avoided is to try to apply more conventional, hierarchical accountability structures to network arrangements. There is clearly a concern among many that networks have become 'uncoupled' from legitimate representatives institutions and, therefore, function on the margins of accountability (see, for example, Rhodes and Wanna 2007: 407). However, the response to this concern should not be to attempt to 'rein in' the network structures, since this would defeat the benefits of network governance in overcoming the fragmentation and disaggregation inherent in modern society. A more productive (and ultimately less futile) approach would be to accept the existence of a 'loose coupling,' of representative institutions and networks (Papadoupolis 2007: 485), combined with broader forms of accountability. In other words, to return to the point made by Aarsæther et al., networks need to be answerable to governmental institutions, and also to their members, and to the public at large.

Related to this is the need to go beyond the rigid distinction between administrative and political accountability. In the traditional model, political accountability rests with elected officials, while non-elected officials are seen as accountable for carrying out the policy direction of their political masters. Without dismissing the important distinction between elected and non-elected officials, public servants are now called upon to play a more proactive role from a policy perspective as a result of their participation in networks. What is needed in the modern world are "public service practitioners who interact with citizens … [and] can take incremental steps toward improving the quality of democracy by actively helping people govern themselves." Finding the appropriate balance between elected and non-elected officials, as well as re-defining appropriate roles for the various actors, will take some time, and no doubt a considerable amount of trial and error. In the short term, it will be important to be open to new possibilities and to integrate a strong learning component into the accountability mechanisms that are developed.

Operating in the 'shadow of hierarchy'

The third question to be addressed concerns whether it is feasible for a network governance model in public health to exist within a larger bureaucratic structure, in this case, the government of Canada, which still operates largely as a traditional hierarchical structure. Granted that network governance operates in the shadow of hierarchy, as Scharf (1994) has stated, one might ask how long is this shadow and to what extent does it permit enough sunlight to allow networked forms of governance to grow?

Kettl rightly points out that "[m]anaging indirect government requires great skill in managing networks, but the existing civil service system was created to manage hierarchies" (Kettl 2002: 499). The problem may be particularly acute in Westminster systems, such as in Canada, with a heavier concentration of power, than in systems with a greater diffusion of power, such as in the United States (Rhodes and Wanna 2007).

There can be little question that the federal public administration in Canada, in theory at least, follows a classic hierarchical structure, with top down command-and-control being the standard way of operating (Gow 2004). Moreover, recent events have tended to 'thicken' this structure. In part, this is related to the government's response to the grants and contributions controversy at the (then called) Department of Human Resources Development Canada (HRDC) in 2000, and more recently the sponsorship affair at Public Works and Government Services Canada in 2004. As discussed in chapter 6, the reaction to these events has led to the creation of new rules intended to increase the scrutiny over public servants and ensure an appropriate level of accountability. To this were added the provisions of the *Federal Accountability Act* of 2006. The unintended cumulative consequence of these changes has been to further reduce the discretion of public servants and to make the public service more rule-driven than has been seen in modern times. The fifth report of the Prime Minister's Advisory Committee on the Public Service specifically expressed concern that the complex reporting requirements that have been introduced over recent years have given rise to "barriers to relationships with many sectors of Canadian society" (Privy Council Office 2011). Unfortunately, this is exactly the opposite of what is needed to make network governance function.

At the same time, there may well be, as Hubbard and Paquet have argued, a significant gap between the "apparent" reality presented by the government, and what is happening "on the ground" (Hubbard and Paquet 2010: 8). Notwithstanding what some have called the 'web of rules,' the complexity of the government of Canada structure is such that innovative practices are still possible as long as one stays 'under the radar.' Although it preceded recent exercises of rules-making, the Canadian Heart Health Initiative, discussed in chapter 5, is an example of an innovative experiment in program design that was deliberately kept from the formal radar screen for fear that official oversight would preclude it from getting off the ground. Although its existence in the margins ultimately led to its demise, the fact that it was able to achieve important results over the course of its twenty-year history is a testimony to the fact that significant activity can and does take place in the bureaucracy outside of the formal rules-based environment. In spite of itself, perhaps, the 'shadow of hierarchy' does allow some rays of light to penetrate.

It may be as well that public health is particularly well positioned to engage in what Paquet has called "scheming virtuously" (Paquet 2009b). As discussed earlier, advocacy is one of the core functions of public health (Chapman 2001). Public health practitioners are trained to see their role as advocating for policies and programs that are conducive to good health. As a part of this, many participate in networks which touch on issues that may or may not be part of government policy. In so doing, they become "virtuous schemers" by virtue of their craft. Because of this, there is a fairly well established tradition in public health of working collaboratively with others outside the hierarchy in which they are located. The example of the Dominion Council of Health was given earlier. In more recent times, McPherson et al. (2007) point out that members of Child Health Networks (CHNs) must learn to "cross-exist" in both traditional hierarchical structures and interorganizational network structures, and to find an appropriate balance between "organizational formalisation and flexibility." As we have seen, it was the attempt to find this balance, in large part, that led to the review and restructuring of the Public Health Network. However, in the absence of a network governance regime – to be discussed in the following chapter – how this balance is struck is bound to be highly variable and, as in the case of the PHN, possibly counterproductive.

Notwithstanding the challenges of attempting to find a place in the hierarchical structures of the formal bureaucracy of the government of Canada, as we saw in our discussion of the PHN, the response to the H1N1 pandemic and the CHHI, there is much to suggest the existence in public health of mechanisms and processes consistent with at least some elements of network governance. Whether conditions exist to allow for the full flourishing of these new models of governance in the current circumstances can only be answered with time. To a certain extent, this will be outside the control of public health practitioners.

What the sector can do, on the other hand, is follow a more conscious and deliberate route to the application of the network governance concept. The next chapter will discuss what steps public health might take to build a public health culture conducive to network governance, as well as to increase its understanding of the basic 'rules of the game' and of the skills and competencies that are needed to apply the concept more consistently and more successfully.

CHAPTER 9

TOWARDS A NETWORK GOVERNANCE REGIME
IN PUBLIC HEALTH

Introduction

This book is essentially a plea for a more conscious, systematic and rigorous application of network governance in the field of public health. Ultimately what is at stake here is more than a little tinkering around the edges. Rather, we refer to the establishment of a network governance regime, a term which Phillips and Graham have defined as "not only ...sets of the rules and relationships among actors, but also of the norms, cultures, and expectations created as a result of these relationships" (Phillips and Graham 2000: 152). This is part of the transition from "Big G" government to "small g" governance (Hubbard and Paquet 2010: 1), which has received a considerable amount of scholarly attention in the literature on public administration and political science. We will argue in this chapter that public health is particularly well-suited to this model of governance, and has the potential to act as somewhat of a vanguard in the application of this concept to the 'real world.'

This is not to suggest that networks and network governance represents some form of organizational panacea. It is undeniable that there are non-trivial risks involved with operationalizing this concept. Case studies have shown that network governance can and often does break down in various circumstances. Furthermore, we have discussed that networks are not necessarily collaborative. Power dynamics can exist within networks that reinforce inequalities and undermine any collaborative aspect

(Kahler 2009: 13). Moreover, there is no ready-made formula to follow for implementation. At most, what can be offered are approaches to reduce the risk of failure, and even those have to be seen as general principles or guidelines, as opposed to hard and fast rules.

On the other hand, the world around us is changing quickly, and will not stop doing so because we are not ready to face the challenges this represents. The better option – perhaps the *only* responsible option – is to explore what these changes mean and how best to adapt to them. There will certainly be obstacles to network governance, so it is best to understand what they are and to seek possible ways to anticipate and, eventually, to overcome them.

Where to from here?

Previous chapters have attempted to demonstrate that there remains a considerable distance to travel before we can speak of a network governance regime in public health. At the national level, the sector has made some positive steps in this direction, and has a number of past and present experiences from which to draw. Yet the steps that have been taken seem tentative, sporadic and disjointed. What is needed at this point is a deliberate and focused strategy to implement network governance by taking concrete steps in this direction and assessing the results of those early activities so that the learnings can be incorporated into future exercises.

The question remains, where to begin? To reiterate, there is no formula to follow in putting network governance into practice. What works in one sector or sub-sector will not necessarily be successful in another. Attempts to provide a list of "success factors" or a recipe for success will at best be overly simplistic and possibly misleading (Huxham and Vangen 2005: 71). In what follows, three broad components will be proposed as "building blocks" for a strategy. They address the need to recognize the nature of the game which is in play, the need to learn the rules of the game, and the need to develop the personal competencies to play the game. Each will be discussed in turn.

1. Recognize the 'game'

The Chief Public Health Officer David Butler-Jones stated in his 2008 report that "it takes the combined effort of networks both within and outside the public health system to address population-wide health challenges" (Public Health Agency of Canada 2008). Yet this must be understood at a deeper level throughout public health organizations, whether at the national, provincial or local levels. What needs to be absorbed within the organizational culture in public health is that network governance is not just a sideline activity – it is rather at the core of how the public health enterprise is conducted, and is relevant to all aspects of public health. The implications of this are far-reaching.

Network governance implies a paradigm shift in how public agencies operate. It is a step in the direction of "authentic public participation," where the public "is part of the deliberation process from issue framing to decision framing" (King et al. 1998: 317). More than requiring new structures and institutions, it represents what some have called a "a full-blown cultural transformation" (Goldsmith and Eggers 2004: 158).[32]

The point is that network governance is a serious concept that needs to be taken seriously. The first step is at the level of awareness that, in this era, the public health business needs to be conducted through networks. Following from this, it is important to apply more rigour to our understanding of what exactly this means. R.A.W. Rhodes points out that too often organizations create "self-steering networks by accident" and do not learn the lessons of how best to steer within these networks (Rhodes 1997: 110). A more analytical approach is necessary in public health to gain a better understanding of which networks are operating in which areas. New tools, such as "network mapping" technologies, are now available to systematically analyze the use and functioning of networks (see for example: Conway 2001; de Nooy et al. 2005). These tools are important in gaining a better understanding of which networks exist in a particular field, whom they include, how they interrelate with each other, what they represent and where to situate the areas of convergence or divergence.

Moreover, it is equally important to know *how* networks operate in terms of inclusiveness, transparency and effectiveness. Such a review may well play a role in determining, for example, whether public health agencies wish to be part of networks that may be weak in some areas, or whether, using the tools of metagovernance, government agencies can help to improve the

[32] Sorensen goes as far as to say that what is implied is nothing less than "a reformulation of the traditional image of liberal democracy" (Sorensen 2002: 715).

functioning of those structures. As part of this, it is important to examine how public health representatives are participating in them, and whether they have the necessary skills and competencies to contribute fully and appropriately to the networks in which they are involved. Since it would be impossible to pursue actively all forms of network involvement simultaneously, an aspect of this approach should also include an assessment of which networks are core to the strategic objectives of the organization. Although, as noted, public health is rich in the area of networks, a careful survey may conclude that networks are lacking in some important areas and that active steps are needed to help establish new ones, or assist in modifying those already in existence.

A key aspect of this analysis should also incorporate the notion that not all networks are the same and that one's participation in or attempts to "metagovern" need to be tailored to the type of network in question. We cited earlier Agranoff's four categories of networks (informational, developmental, outreach and action). In a similar way, Herranz suggests four network management styles along a passive-to-active managerial spectrum which broadly correspond to Agranoff's categories (Herranz 2006: 7). Other categorizations are, of course, possible, but what is important is for public health practitioners to distinguish the types of networks and to assess if the approaches that are being taken to participate in them are the appropriate ones needed for those particular cases.

Finally, while it is important to understand and adjust, as necessary, to the various types of network, it is equally important to realize that they are all networks and as such, share common core characteristics. In chapter 4, we discussed the false dichotomy in public health as seen in the four major reports on the SARS crisis. The view in those reports suggested that a collaborative style of governance was appropriate for some areas in public health, such as health promotion, but that infectious disease emergency response required a hierarchical command-and-control structure. As discussed in that chapter, this view fails to take into account that public health emergencies also call for networked responses, albeit needing a higher level of centralization than in other situations. Although they need to be tailored to specific circumstances, many of the 'rules of the game' of network governance, discussed below, will apply in most circumstances. The first step is to recognize and acknowledge that whether in 'peace-time' or in 'war-time,' public health practitioners need to work with and through networks to accomplish their objectives.

2. Learn the rules of the game

Following from the above, the era of network governance "requires a truly revolutionary collection of strategies and tactics" (Kettl 2002: 508). The essence of network theory is that no single actor can impose its will on others – at least, not for long. Salamon identifies four elements of network theory: what he calls "pluriformity," by which he means the diversity of organizations; self-referentiality, meaning that each organization in a network will have its own interests at heart; asymmetric interdependencies; and dynamism, referring to the constantly changing scene (Salamon 2002: 15). It is clear that this will not be a simple game to play. How, then, does one go about it? The following are proposed as guidelines:

Adjust to the changing role of government

This discussion must begin with the realization that the role of government is no longer what it once was. Several observers have pointed out that we live in a world where no one is in charge, at least not *fully* in charge, or, as others have put it, where "everyone appears to be somewhat in charge"(Paquet 2009b; Hubbard and Paquet 2010; Denhardt and Denhardt 2002: 553; Kettl 2009; Stoker 2006: 52; Agranoff 2007: 191). Kettl's description of current-day society as "(p)luralism on steroids" seems quite apt (Kettl 2009: 11). Government is no longer in a position to simply impose its will on society, based on its interpretation of the public interest. State authorities now need to work with others and, often to empower others, to help define public policy objectives (Posner 2002: 546). As discussed in the previous chapter, government still has a unique role to play, but it must learn to play public policy as a 'team sport.'

This has fundamental implications for how governmental representatives exercise their role. Increasingly, governments are called upon to play a facilitative role, in such a way as to create a space for solutions to come from those most affected by a particular policy or program activity (Denhardt and Denhardt 2002: 553). Furthermore, there is an important role for governments to ensure broad inclusion in a discussion and to go beyond engaging only 'the usual suspects,' that is those groups which have historically been involved with a particular issue and with whom one has an existing relationship. Indeed, government agencies are uniquely placed to see more broadly which other, less obvious, parts of society may have an important stake and ensure that these are also included in the debate.

Finally, to continue with the sporting metaphor, one of the main roles of government is to ensure a 'level playing field,' so that all those who have an interest in an issue, including the more disadvantaged sectors of society, are provided with a real opportunity to participate. The challenge is to find a place "for the involvement of the disorganized many as well as the organized few" (Stoker 2006: 53). This may well mean taking proactive steps to find a place at the table, and providing adequate resources for those elements of society to have a voice in the process.

The sections below will discuss other areas where government can play a key role. Yet the starting point is for government representatives, elected and unelected, to come to terms with the realization (which may not come easily) that they are no longer in complete control and, that to be considered legitimate, the resolution of issues will need to come as a result of the active engagement of the affected parts of society.

Develop a culture of collaboration

Following from above, it is necessary for those working in the public health area, state and non-state, to develop a culture of collaboration within their organizations. In this context, we see culture as referring to the "hidden and largely unquestioned assumptions and beliefs held by members of the organizations that guide their behaviour" (Denhardt and Denhardt 2002: 556). The key part of this culture needs to be the commitment, as stated above, that important public policy decisions need to be made through a process of engagement and deliberation.

This notion requires quite a different mindset on a number of levels. The most obvious is that hierarchy and formal authority are no longer considered sufficient to lend legitimacy to a policy decision. Beyond this, there also needs to be a realization that a purely rational approach to problem solving is no longer appropriate. Such an approach is more typical of new public management, which favours the use of objective standards and indicators to assess efficiency and cost effectiveness. Such measures are undoubtedly still relevant. However, in addition, one needs to include factors that are more subjective, and which reflect an effort to find, through discussion, "a common ground which enables mutual adjustment of strategies and joint action" (Koppenjan and Klijn 2004: 162).

The above point is particularly relevant for a field such as public health which is anchored in scientific methodologies and which strongly values "evidence-based" decision-making. Yet dependence on science, admirable as this may be, may also reveal somewhat of a blind spot in the way in which issues are addressed. Peters has pointed out that "in the end the technical solutions may not always triumph in a complex political environment" (Peters 2007: 72). The way in which research questions are formulated can often reveal biases that widen, rather than narrow differences of perspectives with those who do not share the same perspective (Koppenjan and Klijn 2004: 8). In other words, the research questions one asks and the way one asks them have a major impact on the results. While science and evidence are necessary in a policy discussion, the policy process in the final analysis will be driven by the interests and the perceptions of those participating in the discussion (Kickert and Koppenjan 1997: 54; Box 2002: 29). It is therefore critical to engage stakeholders in the process of framing the research and formulating the research questions for the results to be seen as compelling to the broader community.

There also needs to be a recognition that in order for shared leadership, collaboration and empowerment to become the norm, this governance model must be applied both internally and externally to an organization (Denhardt and Denhardt 2002: 556). An organization which attempts to build external partnerships while functioning in a traditional hierarchical fashion creates an inconsistency which will ultimately undermine its effectiveness. Building a culture of collaboration implies integrating this way of operating in all facets of an organization so that it becomes instinctive for the participants. The patterns of behaviour and competencies which are to be encouraged in dealings with stakeholders and partners must also be applied to the internal environment so that collaboration becomes the *modus operandi* of the organization in question. Because the PHAC and Health Canada are part of the organizational structure of the government of Canada and will, therefore, reflect the hierarchical nature of that structure, developing an organizational culture around a different governance model will be challenging. To a certain extent, this will continue to be the case for public servants generally for some time. Many public servants need to operate in two worlds. On the one hand, they need to work within the parameters of a formal organization, which involves rules, hierarchy, budgets, audits, reviews, authorizations and so on. At the same time, they are asked to perform tasks which are collaborative by nature – negotiating, coordinating, linking, adjusting, and joint problem solving (Agranoff 2007: 197).

Challenging as developing a culture of collaboration within a traditional bureaucratic organization may be, it is a fundamental step to be taken. As Huerta et al. point out: "The failure to inculcate a 'network' culture, within the member organizations, as well as the collective as a whole, results in parallel rather than integrated structures, to the eventual demise of the network" (Huerta et al. 2007: 18). Some areas, however, such as public health, offer the possibility, through incremental steps, to shift the balance over time in favour of a more collaborative model.

Employ the 'right' leadership style

As previously mentioned, network governance does not preclude leadership. Quite the contrary, leadership is a "crucial precondition of success" (Kickert and Koppenjan 1997: 58). What differs from the hierarchical model is the *style* of leadership. Leadership based on hierarchy and rank is clearly not what is required, in fact, such a style can be quite damaging in a network. Rather, what is needed is someone who can lead through influencing others, alternatively encouraging and cajoling. Goldsmith and Eggers refer to a need for 'symphony conductors' rather than 'drill sergeants' (Goldsmith and Eggers 2004: 158). No longer is it the case that the leader needs to find the solution to the challenges faced by the network. Instead, those in leadership positions need to play a facilitative role so that solutions emerge from the interactions of the stakeholders themselves (Reinicke and Deng 2000: 65). The role of network manager becomes "one of mediator and stimulator of interaction and not one of central director" (Koppenjan and Klijn 2004: 11). Huxham and Vangen identify four leadership activities that are appropriate for a collaboration:

- embracing: getting the 'right' members to join;
- empowering: having right infrastructure to enable people to join;

- involving: managing inequality between principal and subsidiary members;
- mobilizing: ensuring all member organizations benefit (Huxham and Vangen 2005: 228).

What is also involved in the network governance context is a notion of shared leadership. This style of leadership focuses on the "goals, values, and ideals that the organization and community want to advance." It must be characterized by mutual respect, accommodation, and support (Denhardt and Denhardt 2002: 167). Consistent with the notion that no one is fully in charge, this type of leadership is not concentrated in one person. Rather, "leaders at various levels play key roles"(Stoker 2006: 52). As seen in the case of the Canadian Heart Health Initiative, too much concentration of leadership on one person, or a very small cadre of individuals, can lead to the premature decline of an initiative if there happens to be a leadership change. A key function in this type of leadership is to fully engage a wide number of individuals, and to foster a sense of empowerment so that all participants feel motivated to contribute fully to achieve the common objective.

This is not to advocate for a passive style of leadership. On the contrary, the leadership role in a network is more time and resource intensive than in a conventional top-down organization, and requires a broader range of skills. Among other factors, what is needed from those in leadership positions is a level of persistence to ensure that a network is not allowed to simply drift along aimlessly. Associated with this is a commitment to action. It is not enough to ensure that people get along. Networks come together for the purpose of achieving a common goal, and success will be predicated on the need to keep focussed on these objectives and to commit to actions that will advance the agenda.

There is also a harder-edged side to network leadership, which can involve having to deal with participants who are not contributing to the collective objectives of the group, or, even worse, who are using the network to achieve their own ends at the expense of others. Huxham and Vangen refer "collaborative thuggery," as the aspect of network leadership which can involve fairly strong methods taken with the objective of advancing the collective agenda (Huxham and Vangen 2005: 79). A network leader may need to move from collaboration to collaborative thuggery as circumstances dictate, or the functions can be moved to other members of the network, depending on need, individual personality traits and other factors. In sum, leadership in network governance requires an understanding of metagovernance, and the tools and competencies to make it work.

Create a learning environment

In the early stages of a network, members will come to the table with knowledge resources that are based on their personal experiences and what they draw from their home organizations. In order to have meaningful conversations, a base for shared knowledge must be established. A good part of the ability to communicate with participants in a network will need to be based on their understanding of each other's views and priorities, and how they have come to these. Those in leadership positions must be prepared to "give away" knowledge and control "to help citizens self-govern" (Box 2002: 34). What is required in this context is an openness to new ideas and approaches and a willingness to share views and information (Stoker 2006: 51). In a scientific area, such as public health, technical learning is obviously necessary. However, it is hardly sufficient. What is also necessary is policy learning, where players develop a better appreciation of the various ways in which a policy issue can be dealt with, as well as a deeper appreciation of the public policy process itself. This is often a necessary step to ensure that the policy issues are framed in a way which responds to the needs and interests of all players and which are more likely to engage a broader cross-section of society. What Huerta et al. observe in health care delivery network models is applicable also in other areas: "Effective HSD [health services delivery] networks require organizational representatives to see beyond the mission of their employing organizations and engage as a multi-organizational participant" (Huerta et al. 2007: 18). This transition is part of the collective learning process. What is key is to foster a commitment to share knowledge and engage in an inclusive process to search for solutions.

Engage in trust building

The importance of trust is a persistent theme in the literature about network governance (i.e., Huxham 2003: Huxham and Vangen 2005; Agranoff 2004: 86; Rhodes 2000: 61; Nelson 2001: 95; Rainey and Busson 2001: 72). Agranoff observes that trust is a network's substitute for mandated authority (Agranoff 2007: 28).

Koppenjan and Klijn argue that "trust is regarded as perception of good intentions of other actors" (Koppenjan and Klijn 2004: 83). Deseve has called it the "glue" of organizations (Deseve 2009: 135). A network in which a level of trust does not manifest itself is unlikely to be able to function effectively for any significant length of time (Imperial 2005: 310).

Yet it is important to recognize that the existence of trust, or perhaps better expressed, the building of trust, should be seen as something that grows out of the relationships that are formed as part of the network, rather than as a pre-condition for the formation of a network. In the early stages, the parties are more likely to be uncertain about how much confidence they can have in the other participants. Most collaborations begin "under a cloud of suspicion" (Huxham and Vangen 2005: 66). Players in a network will often be associated with organizations which are in competition with each other or have a history of friction. This is commonly the case in public health, where VSOs share a common goal of reducing chronic disease, yet are ultimately competing for donations from the public. The same is true, probably more so, with private sector corporations that participate in networks. Governments will also compete with one another to take the credit for an initiative, or alternatively, assign the blame to others for deficiencies or breakdowns. Recognizing that communication will never be fully open, for trust to emerge it is necessary for participants to communicate what motivates and what constrains them (Ibid.: 101). The level of trust builds as participants see that their partners will follow through on their commitments, respect the "turf" of others, and generally act openly and transparently. The process of mutual learning that takes place in a collaboration itself contributes to additional trust (Agranoff 2007: 121). This will, of course, require some time to build, so a certain amount of patience is required as it does so.

It is crucial, therefore, to have *trust building* as a key objective in a collaboration, particularly in its early stages. It is also important to remember that trust builds slowly, but disappears quickly (Koppenjan and Klijn 2004: 231). Parties will need to pay particular attention to following through on their intentions, ensure that their actions are consistent with their statements and, in the event of changes in their positions, ensure that these are communicated clearly to the other members, with appropriate explanations of the reasons for such changes. Changes in the institutional design of networks should also be approached very cautiously, for they can easily set back efforts in trust building (Ibid.: 232).

Apply principles of network design and management

There are several right and wrong ways to design a network. Without attempting to be exhaustive, or overly prescriptive, a number of themes emerge as key to network formation as follows:[33]

Seek commitment to a common purpose or mission. Developing common goals or at least a common agenda is a fundamental step in network formation. There needs to be some sense of what a network wishes to achieve together. What seems like an obvious statement, however, is far from it. Participating organizations and individuals will enter into a network with their own set of preconceived notions of what is important and perceptions of the other actors. Huxham and Vangen observe that collaborative aims exist "in an entanglement of other aims, both real and imagined" (Huxham and Vangen 2005: 74). It is therefore necessary to take the time needed to develop the goals jointly with the other participants and to ensure that they are genuinely committed to those goals. Furthermore, there are two important caveats to consider. First, the objective is not to find a high level of consensus on all points. With a number of diverse players coming to the table with their own organizational and individual aspirations, this is unlikely to occur. It is more realistic to seek "the minimum agreement which allows for joint action" (Termeer and Koppenjan 1997: 87). Provan and Kenis have shown that networks can function quite effectively with only moderate levels of goal consensus, provided that network relationships are well managed (Provan and Kenis 2007: 240). Second, it is important to recognize that this will be a dynamic process, not a static one. In the best of scenarios, it may mean that through a mutual learning process, members will adjust their original goals to more shared targets (Nelson 2001: 91). The practical significance is that as part of the nurturing process discussed below, time will need to be spent to either confirm, adjust, or re-define the purpose bringing the parties together.

Establish criteria for membership. It is obviously important to be inclusive of all different interests related to an issue, particularly if there is a high level of disagreement in a field.

---

[33] For this, we make selective use of the list provided in Deseve's discussion of networks in the intelligence community (Deseve 2009: 135-36).

On the other hand, one can be too inclusive by accepting anyone in the process who has expressed an interest, however remote. While laudable, this can sometimes weigh down the discussions, cause distractions, and dilute the product that the players are working towards. The main players should be those with the greatest interest and with the most to contribute (not necessarily monetarily) to advancing an issue. Network management also includes finding a way to deal with negative behaviours, such as with 'free-riding,' referring to players who may not have much to contribute, or who may choose not to contribute; 'hit and run' strategies, where a member leaves the group as soon as his/her personal or corporate objectives are met; and 'wait and see' approaches, for players who will not commit themselves until they know more about what the end result is likely to be (Koppenjan and Klijn 2004: 51). There can also be members who might have ulterior motives, such as finding out what their 'competition' is doing, or perhaps even seeking to sabotage the network. In other words, network governance, while inclusive, is not a free-for-all, nor can one always assume the best intentions from all parties. A part of metagovernance is to ensure that there is some measure of network discipline within the structure for the network to keep making progress towards its goals. Having members who are there for the wrong reasons, or for no reason, can demoralize those players who are committed to achieving the collective goals, and potentially lead to infighting or loss of valuable contributors. This is one area where 'collaborative thuggery' has an appropriate place.

Establish a dispute resolution mechanism. Although public health is not normally an area in which pitched battles occur, there are inevitably occasions when conflicts arise. We saw in the case of the Canadian Heart Health Initiative that progress was hampered somewhat by the lack of a mechanism to deal with disputes over 'turf.' While Pierre is probably right in saying we do not know yet how to manage conflict in networks successfully (Pierre 2000: 245), it remains important to have mechanisms in place, whether formal or informal, to address openly issues causing conflicts, rather than letting them fester and potentially interfering with the workings of the network. The mechanisms can be adapted or changed if they prove ineffective, but it is important to have something on which to build and to learn.

Maintain access to authority. It was stated earlier that network governance exists in the 'shadow of hierarchy,' and needs to exist in reality as a complex blend of vertical and horizontal management. Without adopting a top-down management model, there are critical points where formal authority needs to be brought into the picture. As an example, one of the reasons for the premature demise of the Canadian Heart Health Initiative was that it was, in fact, too successful at keeping 'under the radar,' and had no defenders among senior decision makers when the continuation of its resource base became vulnerable.

Secure adequate resources. The resource needs, both human and financial, will vary according to what the network wishes to accomplish, but some level of resourcing will inevitably be required.

Share information freely. In networks, "empowerment is based on information rather than authority" (Agranoff 2007: 27). While the level of intensity of interaction might vary according to the nature of the network, most networks are largely in the knowledge management business (Ibid.: 29). Network members will expect to be kept informed of new developments in their area of interest, in particular as it relates to the public policy process. How is the government of the day dealing with their issue? Are there international developments that might have an impact on how the issue will be handled domestically? What are the activities that some members are conducting that the other members could learn from? In addition, members will want to be kept apprised of new research that has a bearing on their area of interest. Without regular communications among the members, a network exists in name only.

Modern communications technology has had a huge impact in the development of network governance. At least one observer has posited that the "emerging information or knowledge era makes collaborative networking imperative" (Ibid.: 156). This is so for two reasons. First, modern technology has made information much more widely accessible than before. This has led to an increased number of participants who have left the stands and are now on the field and expecting to play in the game, to extend the metaphor used by Denhardt and Denhardt. It is no longer possible, therefore, for information to be controlled by any one actor (Ibid.: 101). Second, because of the sheer volume of information that is now available and, because much of it is so specialized, no single participant can realistically claim to absorb and comprehend all of it. This then leads to dependence on others to be able to translate the information that is available into knowledge that is useful to further the objectives of a particular network.

Modern communications has therefore democratized the access to information and increased the reliance of stakeholders on each other in the use of this information, both of which have significant benefits from a network governance perspective. Timely circulation of information keeps members up to date on developments, contributes to policy and technical learning and helps to build trust among the members.

Nurture...selectively

Huxham and Vangen stress the need to "nurture, nurture, nurture" (Huxham and Vangen 2005: 42). Many things can go wrong within networks, and it is impossible to anticipate every one. The best prescription to avoid governance failure in networks is "conscious and careful network management" (Sorensen and Torfing 2007: 102). Network managers need to invest time and attention if they expect a network to produce positive results. Comparing nurturing a network to tending a garden, Huxham and Vangen point out that there will be times when only light effort will be sufficient, and others when major weeding and pruning will be necessary. In both cases, the conclusion is that, much like tending a garden, a network must continuously be nurtured.

The necessary corollary for this is that the network manager will need to be realistic about how many networks she/he can lead, and be selective about which ones to take on. Public health practitioners are regularly faced with requests to lead, or otherwise participate in, networks on a host of issues. This can easily lead to unsustainable situations where the individual involved is simply not able to provide the necessary attention to deal with the myriad issues that will surface in the course of a network. As Director General of the Centre for Health Promotion at the PHAC, this author was a participant, often as chair or co-chair, of literally dozens of networks, and found that giving each the time and attention it warranted was completely unsustainable. It is necessary to assess at the outset which networks are most closely related to the strategic objectives of the organization to which one belongs, and to make decisions about participation on that basis. Moreover, reassessments must be made on a regular basis, since there is a tendency to 'accumulate' networks in which one participates. Priorities and circumstances change, as does the strategic value of any particular network. These developments have implications for decisions about where to put one's efforts. Decisions about changes of direction, however, need to be made with due attention to the impact such changes could have on relationships with other participants.

Make strategic use of incentives

Collaborative ventures often fail due to fear, lack of ambition, risk aversion and the power of negative incentives (Perri 6 et al.: 2002: 124). This may be particularly problematic in traditional hierarchies, where risk-taking is not encouraged, and often punished. Moreover, there is sometimes a tendency for some to suspect those in their organizations who participate in networks of colluding with outside parties and, therefore, of not being altogether trustworthy. Less ominously, working within networks is often somewhat invisible, and the supervisors of network participants may not have a good understanding of the contribution their employees are making. To counter this, well conceived incentives must be put in place in the organization to encourage behaviour patterns conducive to participating in networks in a positive and constructive manner (Goldsmith and Eggers 2004: 131).

Avoid perfectionism

Decision making by a significant number of players with different backgrounds, perspectives and priorities is bound to be challenging to even the most skilled and experienced. It can be taken as a given that the final product, whatever it is, will not reflect exactly the views of everyone. What must be encouraged is an approach that "good-enoughism" will lead to far more production and far fewer conflicts, than a culture of perfectionism (Huxham and Vangen 2005: 257). Players need to remember that "the perfect is the enemy of the good" (Goldsmith and Eggers 2004: 180).

Strike the balance between process and action

Much of the previous discussion revolved around process elements related to making collaborations work effectively. At the same time, it is important to ensure that the action goals of the network are not overlooked. Again, depending on the type of network, those goals will differ, as will the means of achieving them. But the risk of "collaborative inertia" is everpresent. It is entirely conceivable that in an effort to ensure all points of view are aired and getting equal attention, a collaboration can be turned into a "talking shop" with very few achievements to show (Stoker 2006: 56). What is needed is a careful balance between the two. As Wadell and Brown put it: "A single-minded focus upon process can paralyze a partnership in endless repetitive discussions, while a single-minded focus upon product can blow it apart" (Wadell and Brown 1997: 23). Finding an appropriate balance between those two elements will be a function of attentiveness and good judgment.

Use technology...appropriately

Modern technology has dramatically changed the environment for networks. Sharing information to almost any point in Canada, or for that matter, around the world, can be done instantly and at almost no cost. It is also possible for meetings to be held 'virtually,' thus saving both time and money for the participants. Social media technology opens many new opportunities that were not available before the last few decades. At the same time, however, too much dependence on technology can be damaging. Face-to-face contact, to some extent, remains necessary to allow network partners to develop personal relationships, build trust and communicate effectively (Goldsmith and Eggers 2004: 96). It also needs to be recognized that different techniques and technologies are necessary depending on whether one is dealing with a small group (25 and under), a large mass (over 100,000), or, as will most often be the case, a point in between (Wilson 2011).

3. Develop the personal competencies to play the game

Understanding the game one is in and the 'rules' about how to play it, while necessary, are both necessary but not sufficient to playing the game well. What is also necessary is to acquire the skills to play the game. McPherson et al., in their review of child health networks, are quite right in suggesting that although members are committed to collaboration, unless they are aware of how to operate in network structures and have the skills to do so, they will "continue to construct traditional policies and management techniques characteristic of traditional public service sectors." (McPherson et al. 2007: 50). Unfortunately, there is no network governance equivalent to POSDCORB – planning, organizing, staffing, directing, coordinating, reporting, budgeting – associated with hierarchical management (Agranoff and McGuire 2003: 1403). Nevertheless, there is a considerable amount of convergence in the literature about the types of skills that are required in collaborative governance. Kettl, for instance, identifies five skills needed: goal setting, negotiation, communication, financial management and bridge building (Kettl 2002: 504). Goldsmith and Eggers, for their part, list: negotiation, mediation, risk analysis, trust building, collaboration, project management, strategic thinking, interpersonal communicating, team building, and project and business management (Goldsmith and Eggers 2004: 158). Waddell and Brown include: trust building; integrating multiple perspectives, negotiating power and resources differences; identifying common ground; and creating shared visions (Waddell and Brown 1997: 2). Salamon uses a different language to get at much the same types of competencies in identifying four elements needed for network governance:

- enablement skills, referring to the ability to engage partners and bring multiple stakeholders together for a common cause;
- activation skills, the ability to find appropriate partners and identify new opportunities;
- orchestration skills, which includes enabling, coordinating, and persuading, and project management; and
- modulating skills, meaning finding the right combination of incentives and penalties (Salamon 2002: 16-7).

Drawing from this literature, one sees a combination of two sets of competencies. The first are what might be called the interpersonal skills – the 'soft' skills – relating to communication, negotiation, trust building, facilitation, mediation and conflict resolution. The second category refers to the somewhat sharper-edged business management skills involving such matters as risk analysis, budgeting and project coordination. It is not necessary that individuals participating in networks have both sets of skills, but the network collectively needs to have capacity at both levels.

To the above lists should also be added the ability to progress in an environment characterized by ambiguity and complexity (Huxham and Vangen 2005: 72). This may be particularly relevant to public health practitioners. As we have discussed, the fragmentation and overlapping nature of public health are such that it is important to see the interconnections between issues, without becoming stymied by the complexity that emerges therefrom. Nor does one have the luxury to wait until irrefutable evidence becomes available to prescribe every step that must be taken. Science does not trump judgment. For the foreseeable future, public health leaders will need to continue to operate in a world where certainty is unobtainable and where they must continue to draw conclusions on the basis of incomplete or even contradictory information.

Finally, a critical competency is the ability to engage in what Stoker has called "the role of reflection, lesson drawing and continuous adaptation" (Stoker 2006: 49). This skill involves engaging in retrospective analysis and learning. Because so much of network governance is yet to be adequately studied and understood, it is important to invest the time and resources in analyzing and documenting insights drawn from participation in various processes. Although process considerations can sometimes be seen as being secondary, particularly in science-based sectors, it is important to apply the same type of rigour to process considerations as is applied to the substantive elements of the issues involved. In other words, it is not strictly a question of "results achieved" that must be examined, but also 'path taken.' This means building the capacity to be self-conscious and self-analytical about what was attempted, what resulted, and what can and should be adapted in the future. Since objective criteria are still lacking in many instances, case studies are a particularly useful tool. But whatever tool one uses, the critical factor is to develop and maintain the discipline to regularly and systematically draw learnings from previous experience and apply them to current and future processes.

Conclusion

While the three steps proposed above – recognizing the game one is in, learning the ground rules, and acquiring the skills to play the game – lead to fundamental changes for how to manage the public health enterprise, they can be approached modestly and incrementally. An enhanced appreciation of the fact that advances in public health, whether in emergency or non-emergency situations, is dependent on participation in networks, in and of itself represents a significant step. This is particularly the case if it leads to a more systematic assessment of the networks in which one is already participating and which of these is of greatest strategic importance. Similarly, a stronger focus on the basic elements to make network participation more fruitful, accompanied by steps to enhance appropriate competencies within public health agencies will require some time to bear fruit, but can be carried out in a step-by-step fashion.

The complexities of modern society have led to a search for new approaches to governance. New tools are needed to deal more effectively with the 'wicked problems' that challenge liberal-democratic systems. It is in this context that one can understand the high level of interest in network governance over the past few decades. It is indeed the case that networks "have become the intellectual enterprise of our era" (Kahler 2009: 2).

As has been stressed throughout this book, public health is well positioned to take a leadership role in developing the new tools, mechanisms and competencies that are needed. The long experience public health has had in working with a large and diverse array of stakeholders and, of attempting to do so in a collaborative fashion, provides a rich basis from which to draw a better understanding of the mechanisms and practices that are most effective in particular circumstances. Similarly, the network infrastructure which currently exists in the area, though imperfect, can be a platform for a more rigorous and consistent approach to network governance.

To a certain extent, this journey has already begun. At the same time, it seems clear that much more needs to be done. To use the quite prominent example of the Public Health Network, as was seen earlier, this initiative represents a fairly sophisticated piece of network infrastructure, particularly from an intergovernmental perspective. At the same time, however, hierarchy, control and exclusivity remain quite prominent in the PHN, and the recent changes to it have made them more so. What is needed now, not solely related to the PHN but to be applied to the many theatres in which public health operates, is a deeper appreciation of what network governance entails, and how best to 'metagovern' in a networked world.

One of the clear conclusions that can be drawn from the theoretical and case study literature is that network governance is not a 'paint-by-numbers' process. It must be adjusted to suit the circumstances in which it is applied, which requires knowledge, judgment and creativity. A great deal must yet be learned about how best to make these adjustments. The complex and fragmented policy environment around public health in Canada puts it in an excellent position to benefit from and contribute to this global conversation. It is an opportunity not to be missed.

BIBLIOGRAPHY

6, Perri, Diana Leat, Kimberly Seltzer and Gerry Stoker. 2002. *Towards Holistic Governance: The New Reform Agenda.* Hampshire, UK: Palgrave.

Aarsæther, Nils, Hilde Bjorna, Trine Fotel and Eva Sorensen. 2009. "Evaluating the Democratic Accountability of Governance Networks: Analysing Two Nordic Megaprojects," *Local Government Studies,* 35(5): 577-594.

Agranoff, Robert. 2004. "Leveraging Networks: A Guide for Public Managers Working Across Organizations" in *Collaboration: Using Networks and Partnerships.* John M. Kamensky and Thomas J. Burlin (eds.). Lanham, MD: Rowman and Littlefield, p. 62-102.

Agranoff, Robert. 2007. *Managing Within Networks.* Washington, DC: Georgetown University Press.

Agranoff, Robert and Michael McGuire. 2003. "Integrating the Paradigms of Intergovernmental and Network Management," *International Journal of Public Administration,* 26(12): 1401-1422.

Angus, Douglas E. and Monique Bégin. 2000. "Governance in Health Care: Dysfunctions and Challenges" in *Governance in the 21ˢᵗ Century: Transactions of the Royal Society of Canada.* Gilles Paquet and David M. Hayne (eds.). Toronto: University of Toronto Press, p. 171-93.

Annan, Kofi. 2006. Secretary General's opening address to the fifty-third annual Department of Public Information/NGO conference, February 22-23. http://www.un.org/dpi/ngosection/annualconfs/53/sg-address.html.

Ansell, Chris and Alison Gash. 2008. "Collaborative Governance in Theory and Practice," *Journal of Public Administration Research and Theory*, 18(4): 543-571.

Armstrong, Jim and Donald G. Lenihan. 1999. *From Controlling to Collaborating: When Governments Want to be Partners*. Toronto: Institute of Public Administration of Canada.

Atkinson, Michael M. and William D. Coleman. 1992. "Policy Networks, Policy Communities and the Problems of Governance," *International Journal of Policy and Administration*, 5(2): 154-180.

Bakvis, Herman and Luc Juillet. 2004. *The Horizontal Challenge: Line Departments, Central Agencies, and Leadership*. Ottawa: Canada School of Public Service.

Bangkok Charter for Health Promotion in a Globalized World. 2005. 6th Global Conference on Health Promotion, Bangkok, Thailand, August.

Banting, Keith G. (ed.). 2000. *The Nonprofit Sector in Canada: Roles and Responsibilities*. Montreal and Kingston: McGill-Queen's University Press.

Benner, Thorsten, Wolfgang H. Reinicke and Jan Martin Witte. 2003. "Global Policy Networks: Lessons Learned and Challenges Ahead," *Brookings Review*, 21(2): 18-22.

Bernier, Nicole and Nathalie Burlone. 2007. "Breaking the Deadlock: Public Health Policy Coordination as the Next Step," *Healthcare Policy*, 3(2): 1-11.

Blue Ribbon Panel on Grant and Contribution Programs. 2006. *From Red Tape to Clear Results*. Ottawa: Government of Canada.

Bogason, Peter and Juliet Musso. 2006. "The Democratic Prospects of Network Governance," *American Review of Public Administration*, 36(1): 3-18.

Bogason, Peter, Sandra Kensen and Hugh T. Miller. 2002. "Pragmatic, Extra-Formal Democracy," *Administrative Theory & Praxis*, 24(4): 675-692.

Boin, Arjen and Paul 't Hart. 2003. "Public Leadership in times of Crisis: Mission Impossible?" *Public Administration Review*, 63(5): 544-553.

Boris, Elizabeth T. and C. Eugene Steuerle (eds.). 1999. *Non-Profits and Government: Collaboration and Conflict.* Washington, DC: The Urban Institute Press.

Börzel, Tanja A. 1998. "Organizing Babylon – On the Different Conceptions of Policy Networks," *Public Administration,* 76 (summer): 253-273.

Börzel, Tanja A. and Diana Panke. 2007. "Network Governance: Effective and Legitimate?" in *Theories of Democratic Network Governance.* Eva Sorensen and Jacob Torfing (eds.). New York: Palgrave Macmillan, p. 153-166.

Bovens, Mark, Thomas Schillemans and Paul 't Hart. 2008. "Does Public Accountability Work? An Assessment Tool," *Public Administration,* 86(1): 225-242.

Box, Richard C., Gary S. Marshall, B.J. Reed and Christine M. Reed. 2001. "New Public Management and Substantive Democracy," *Public Administration Review,* 61(5): 608-619.

Box, Richard C. 2002. "Pragmatic Discourse and Administrative Legitimacy," *American Review of Public Administration,* 32(1): 20-39.

Braën, André. 2002. *Health and the Distribution of Powers in Canada.* Ottawa: Commission on the Future of Health Care in Canada. Discussion Paper no. 2.

British Columbia. 2009. *Mobilizing Intersectoral Action to Promote Health: The Case of ActNowBC.* Victoria: Government of British Columbia.

Broadbent Report. 1999. See *Building on Strength: Improving Governance and Accountability in Canada's Voluntary Sector.*

Brock, Kathy. 2001. "Democracy is Coming: The New Interest in NGOs, Civil Society and the Third Sector," *The Philanthropist,* 16(4): 263-271.

Brock, Kathy L. 2004. "Judging the VSI: Reflections on the Relationship between the Federal Government and the Voluntary Sector," *The Philanthropist,* 19(3): 168-181.

Brock, Kathy L. and Associates. 2007. *Measuring the Impact of Voluntary Health Organizations.* Unpublished paper presented to the Office of the Voluntary Sector: Centre for Health Promotion, Public Health Agency of Canada.

Building on Strength: Improving Governance and Accountability in Canada's Voluntary Sector (Broadbent Report). 1999. Prepared by the Panel on Accountability and Governance in the Voluntary Sector.

Butler-Jones, David. 2009. "Public Health Science and Practice: From Fragmentation to Alignment," *Canadian Journal of Public Health,* 100(1): I1-2.

Butterfoss, Frances Dunn, Robert M. Goodman and Abram Wandersman. 1993. "Community Coalitions for Prevention and Health Promotion," *Health Education Research,* 8(3): 315-330.

Campbell Report. 2004. See SARS Commission, *Interim Report.*

Campbell Report. 2005a. See SARS Commission, *Second Interim Report.*

Campbell Report. 2005b. See SARS Commission, *Final Report.*

Cameron, David and Richard Simeon. 2002. "Intergovernmental Relations in Canada: The Emergence of Collaborative Federalism," *Publius: The Journal of Federalism,* 32(2): 49-71.

Canada-US Pan-Border Public Health Preparedness Council, www.pbphpc.org.

Canadian Institutes for Health Research (Institute on Population and Public Health). 2003. "The Future of Public Health in Canada: Developing a Public Health System for the 21st Century." Unpublished report.

Canadian Medical Association. 2003a. *CMA Submission on Infrastructure and Governance of the Public Health System.* Presentation to the Senate Standing Committee on Social Affairs, Science and Technology, October 8.

Canadian Medical Association. 2003b. *Answering the Call.* Submission to the National Advisory Committee on SARS and Public Health, June 25.

Canadian Strategy for Cancer Control. 2006. *A Cancer Plan for Canada.* Discussion Paper. www.partnershipagainstcancer.ca, July.

Cannon, Geoffrey. 2004. "Why the Bush Administration and the Global Sugar Industry are Determined to Demolish the 2004 WHO Global Strategy on Diet, Physical Activity and Health," *Public Health Nutrition,* 7(3): 369-380.

Centres for Disease Control and Prevention. 2004. "Basic Information about SARS." Fact sheet, January 14.

Chambers, Larry W. and Shannon M. Sullivan. 2007. "Reflections on Canada's Public Health Enterprise in the 21st Century," *Healthcare Papers,* 7(3): 22-30.

Chapman, Simon. 2001. "Advocacy in Public Health: Roles and Challenges," *International Epidemiological Association,* 30: 1226-1232.

Clark, Ian D. and Harry Swain. 2005. "Distinguishing the Real from the Surreal in Management Reform: Suggestions for Beleaguered Administrators in the Government of Canada," *Canadian Public Administration,* 48(4): 453-476.

Cleveland, Harlan. 1985. "The Twilight of Hierarchy: Speculations on the Global Information Society," *Public Administration Review,* 45(1): 185-195.

Coleman, William D. and Grace Skogstad. 1990. *Policy Communities and Policy Networks: A Structural Approach.* Toronto: Copp Clark Pitman.

Collin, Jeff. 2004. "Tobacco Politics," *Development,* 47(2): 91-96.

Collin, Jeff, Kelley Lee and Karen Bissell. 2005. "Negotiating the Framework Convention on Tobacco Control: An Updated Politics of Global Health Governance" in *The Global Governance Reader.* Rorden Wilkinson (ed.). London and New York: Routledge, p. 252-273.

Commission on Global Governance. 2005. "A New World" in *The Global Governance Reader.* Rorden Wilkinson (ed.). London and New York: Routledge, p. 26-44.

Commission on the Social Determinants of Health. 2008. *Closing the Gap in a Generation: Health Equity Through Action on the Social Determinants of Health.* Geneva: World Health Organization.

Conference of Principal Investigators of Heart Health. 2002. *Canadian Heart Health Initiative: Process Evaluation of the Demonstration Phase.* Ottawa: Health Canada.

Conway, Steve. 2001. "Employing Social Network Mapping to Reveal Tensions Between Informal and Formal Organisations" in *Social Interaction and Organizational Change*. Oswald Jones, Steve Conway, and Fred Steward (eds.). London, UK: Imperial College Press, p. 81-124.

Corber, Stephen. 2007. "A Dynamic and Ever-Expanding Agenda," *Healthcare Papers*, 7(3): 37-43.

Deber, Raisa, Christopher McDougall and Kumanan Wilson. 2007. "Public Health Through a Different Lens," *Healthcare Papers*. 7(3): 66-71.

Delaney, Faith G. 1994. "Muddling through the Middle Ground: Theoretical Concerns in Intersectoral Collaboration and Health Promotion," *Health Promotion International*, 9(13): 217-225.

deLeon, Peter, and Danielle M. Varda. 2009. "Toward a Theory of Collaborative Policy Networks: Identifying Structural Tendencies," *The Policy Studies Journal*, 37(1): 59-74.

Denhardt Robert B. and Janet V. Denhardt. 2000. "The New Public Service: Serving Rather than Steering," *Public Administration Review* 60(6): 549-559.

Denhardt Janet V. and Robert B. Denhardt. 2002. *The New Public Service: Serving, Not Steering*. Armonk, NY: M.E. Sharpe.

de Nooy, Wouter, Andrej Mrvar and Vladimir Batagelj. 2005. *Exploratory Social Network Analysis with Pajek*. Cambridge, UK: Cambridge University Press.

Deseve, G. Edward. 2009. "'Integration and Innovation' in the Intelligence Community: The Role of a Netcentric Environment, Managed Networks, and Social Networks" in *Unlocking the Power of Networks: Keys to High-Performance Government*. Stephen Goldsmith and Donald F. Kettl (eds.). Washington, DC: Brookings Institution Press, p. 121-144.

de Tocqueville, Alexis. 1945. *Democracy in America*. New York: Vintage Books.

Dodgson, Richard, Kelley Lee and Nick Drager. 2002. "Global Health Governance: A Conceptual Review." Discussion Paper no. 1. London, UK: London School of Hygiene & Tropical Medicine/World Health Organization.

Drabek, Thomas E. and David A. McEntire. 2003. "Emergent Phenomena and the Sociology of Disaster: Lessons, Trends and Opportunities from the Research Literature," *Disaster Prevention and Management*, 12(2): 97-112.

Dupré, Stefan J. 1987. "The Workability of Executive Federalism in Canada" in *Federalism and the Role of the State*. Herman Bakvis and William M. Chandler (eds.). Toronto: University of Toronto Press, p. 236-258.

"Editorial." 2009. *Canadian Medical Journal*, August 17.

Elliott, S.J., S.M. Taylor, R. Cameron and R. Schabas. 1998. "Assessing Public Health Capacity to Support Community-based Heart Health Promotion: The Canadian Heart Health Initiative, Ontario Project (CHHIOP)," *Health Education Research Theory and Practice*, 13(4): 602-622.

Epp, (The Hon.) Jake. 1987. "Achieving Health for All (*The Epp Report*)," *Health Promotion*, 1(4): 419-28.

Expert Panel on SARS and Infectious Disease Control (*Walker Report*). 2004. Final Report. Toronto: Government of Ontario.

Federal/Provincial Working Group on the Prevention and Control of Cardiovascular Disease. 1987. *Promoting Heart Health in Canada*. Ottawa: Health and Welfare Canada.

Fidler, David P. 2003. "SARS: Political Pathology of the First Post-Westphalian Pathogen," *Journal of Law, Medicine & Ethics*, 31: 485-505.

Fidler, David P. 2004a. *SARS, Governance and the Globalization of Disease*. Hampshire, UK: Palgrave Macmillan.

Fidler, David P. 2004b. "Germs, Governance, and Global Public Health in the Wake of SARS," *The Journal of Clinical Investigation*, 113(6): 799-804.

Fidler, David P. 2007. "Reflections on the Revolution in Health and Foreign Policy," *Bulletin of the World Health Organization*, 85(3): 243-244.

Fierlbeck, Katherine. 2010. "Public Health and Collaborative Governance," *Canadian Public Administration*, 53(1): 1-19.

Fischer, Frank. 2003. "Beyond Empiricism: Policy Analysis as Deliberative Practice" in *Deliberative Policy Analysis: Understanding Governance in the Network Society*. Maartin A. Hajer and Hendrick Wagenaar (eds.). Cambridge, UK: Cambridge University Press, p. 209-227.

Flyvbjerg, Bent. 2006. "Five Misunderstandings About Case-Study Research," *Qualitative Inquiry*, 12(2): 219-245.

Gabris, Gerald T. 2004. "Developing Public Managers into Credible Public Leaders: Theory and Practical Implications," *International Journal of Organization Theory and Behavior*, 7(2): 209-231.

Gerth, H.H. and C. Wright Mills (eds.). 1946. *From Max Weber: Essays in Sociology*. New York: Oxford University Press.

Gibson, Kerri, Susan O'Donnell and Vanda Rideout. 2008. "The Project-Funding Regime: Complications for Community Organizations and their Staff," *Canadian Public Administration*, 50(3): 411-435.

Goldsmith, Stephen and William D. Eggers. 2004. *Governing by Network*. Washington, DC: Brookings Institution Press.

Government of Ontario. 2009. *Building Capacity for Local Public Health in Ontario: A Discussion Paper*. Toronto: Ministry of Health and Long-Term Care, Public Health Division.

Gow, Iain. 2004. *A Canadian Model of Public Administration?* Ottawa: Canada School of Public Service.

Grieve, Malcolm. 2003. "Nonprofit Organizations in the Canadian Breast Cancer Network" in *The Nonprofit Sector in Interesting Times: Case Studies in a Changing Sector*. Kathy L. Brock and Keith G. Banting (eds.). Montreal and Kingston: McGill-Queen's University Press, p. 99-128.

Haas, Peter M. 1992. "Introduction: Epistemic Communities and International Policy Coordination," *International Organization*, 46(1): 1-35.

Hajer, Maarten A. 2003. "A Frame in the Fields: Policymaking and the Reinvention of Politics" in *Deliberative Policy Analysis: Understanding Governance in the Network Society*. Maarten A. Hajer and Hendrik Wagernaar (eds.). Cambridge, UK: Cambridge University Press, p. 88-112.

Hajer, Maarten A. and Hendrik Wagernaar. 2003. "Introduction" in *Deliberative Policy Analysis: Understanding Governance in the Network Society*. Maarten A. Hajer and Hendrik Wagernaar (eds.). Cambridge, UK: Cambridge University Press, p. 1-32.

Hall, Michael H., Cathy W. Farr, M. Easwaramoorthy, S. Wojciech Sokolowski and Lester M. Salamon. 2005. *The Canadian Nonprofit and Voluntary Sector in Comparative Perspective*. Toronto: Imagine Canada.

Hardin, Garrett. 1968. "The Tragedy of the Commons," *Science*, 162: 1243-1248.

Hayward, Sarah. 2007. "Networks: Better Language Required," *Healthcare Papers*, 7(2): 62-66.

Health Canada. 1992. *Canadian Heart Health Initiative*. Ottawa: Health Canada.

Health Canada. 2002. *Canadian Heart Health Initiative: Process Evaluation of the Demonstration Phase*. Conference of Principal Investigators of Heart Health. Ottawa: Health Canada.

Health and Welfare Canada. 1987. *Promoting Heart Health in Canada*. Federal/Provincial Working Group on the Prevention and Control of Cardiovascular Disease. Ottawa: Health and Welfare Canada.

Herranz, Joaquin Jr. 2006. *Network Management Strategies*. Evans School working papers series. Seattle, Washington.

Hertting, Nils. 2007. "Mechanisms of Governance Network Formation – A Contextual Rational Choice Perspective" in *Theories of Democratic Network Governance*. Eva Sorenson and Jacob Torfing (eds.). New York: Palgrave Macmillan, p. 43-60.

Hirst, Paul. 2000. "Democracy and Governance" in *Debating Governance: Authority, Steering, and Democracy*. Jon Pierre (ed.). Oxford, UK: Oxford University Press.

Howlett, Michael, M. Ramesh and Anthony Perl. 2009. *Studying Public Policy: Policy Cycles and Policy Subsystems*. 3rd ed. Don Mills, ON: Oxford University Press.

Hubbard, Ruth and Gilles Paquet. 2007. *Gomery's Blinders and Canadian Federalism*. Ottawa: University of Ottawa Press.

Hubbard, Ruth and Gilles Paquet. 2010. *The Black Hole of Public Administration*. Ottawa: University of Ottawa Press.

Huerta, Timothy R., Ann Casebeer and Madine VanderPlaat. 2007. "Using Networks to Enhance Health Services Delivery: Perspectives, Paradoxes and Propositions," *Healthcare Papers*, 7(2): 10-25.

Huxham, Chris. 2003. "Theorizing Collaboration Practice," *Public Management Review*, 5(3): 401-423.

Huxham, Chris and Siv Vangen. 2000. "Leadership in the Shaping and Implementation of Collaboration Agendas: How Things Happen in a (Not Quite) Joined-Up World," *Academy of Management Journal*, 43(6): 1159-1175.

Huxham, Chris and Siv Vangen. 2005. *Managing to Collaborate: The Theory and Practice of Collaborative Advantage*. London and New York: Routledge.

Imagine Canada. 2007a. *Value Added: The Impact of Canada's Charities and Non-Profits*. Toronto: Imagine Canada.

Imagine Canada. 2007b. "Greater than the Sum of Our Parts." Voluntary Sector Awareness Project. Toronto: Imagine Canada.

Imagine Canada. 2011. "Election Kit 2011." Toronto: Imagine Canada.

Imperial, Mark T. 2005. "Using Collaboration as a Governance Strategy: Lessons from Six Watershed Management Programs," *Administration & Society*, 37(3): 281-320.

Innes, Judith E. and David E. Booher. 2003. "Collaborative Policy-making: Governance Through Dialogue" in *Deliberative Policy Analysis: Understanding Governance in the Network Society*. Maarten A. Hajer and Hendrick Wagenaar (eds.). Cambridge, UK: Cambridge University Press, p. 33-54.

Integrated Pan-Canadian Healthy Living Strategy, 2005. Ottawa: Public Health Agency of Canada.

Jackman, M. 2000. "Constitutional Jurisdiction over Health in Canada," *Health Law Journal*, 8: 95-117.

Jackson, Edward T. 2010. "Regrouping, Recalibrating, Reloading: Strategies for Financing Civil Society in Post-Recession Canada," *The Philanthropist*, 23(2): 359-368.

Johns, Carolyn M., Patricia L. O'Reilly and Gregory J. Inwood. 2006. "Intergovernmental Innovation and the Administrative State in Canada," *Governance: An International Journal of Policy, Administration, and Institutions*, 19 (4): 627-649.

Jones, Candace, William S. Hesterly and Stephen P. Borgatti. 1997. "A General Theory of Network Governance: Exchange Conditions and Social Mechanisms," *Academy of Management Review*, 22(4): 911-945.

Juillet, Luc, Caroline Andrew, Tim Aubry and Janet Mrenica. 2001. "The Impact of Changes in the Funding Environment on Nonprofit Organizations" in *The Nonprofit Sector and Government in a New Century*. Kathy L. Brock and Keith G. Banting (eds.). Montreal and Kingston: McGill-Queen's University Press, p. 21-62.

Kahler, Miles (ed.). 2009. *Networked Politics: Agency, Power, and Governance*. Ithaca, NY and London, UK: Cornell University Press.

Kamensky, John M., Thomas J. Burlin and Mark A. Abramson. 2004. "Networks and Partnerships: Collaborating to Achieve Results No One Can Achieve Alone" in *Collaboration: Using Networks and Partnerships*. John M. Kamensky and Thomas J. Burlin (eds.). Lanham, MD: Rowman and Littlefield, p. 3-20.

Keelan, Jennifer. 2008. "Concurrency in Public Health Governance: The Case of the National Immunization Strategy," Special Series: The Role of Federalism in Protecting the Public's Health. Kingston, ON: Institute of Intergovernmental Relations, Queen's University.

Keelan, Jennifer, Harvey Lazar and Kumanan Wilson. 2008. "The National Immunization Strategy: A Model for Resolving Jurisdictional Disputes in Public Health," *Canadian Journal of Public Health*, 99(5): 376-379.

Kettl, Donald F. 2000. "The Transformation of Governance: Globalization, Devolution, and the Role of Government," *Public Administration Review*, 60(6): 488-497.

Kettl, Donald F. 2002. "Managing Indirect Government" in *The Tools of Government: A Guide to the New Government*. Lester M. Salamon (ed.). Oxford, UK: Oxford University Press, p. 490-510.

Kettl, Donald F. 2009. "The Key to Networked Government" in *Unlocking the Power of Networks: Keys to High-Performance Government*. Stephen Goldsmith and Donald F. Kettl (eds.). Washington, DC: Brookings Institution Press, p. 1-14.

Khator, Renu and Nicole A. Brunson. 2001. "Creating Networks for Interorganizational Settings: A Two-Year Follow-up Study in Determinants" in *Getting Results Through Collaboration*. Myrna P. Mandell (ed.). Westport, CT: Quorum Books, p. 154-166.

Kickbusch, Ilona, Gaudenz Silberscmidt and Paulo Buss. 2007. "Global Health Diplomacy: The Need for New Perspectives, Strategic Approaches and Skills in Global Health," *Bulletin of the World Health Organization*, 85(3): 230-232.

Kickert, W.J.M. and Joop F.M. Koppenjan. 1997. "Public Management and Network Management: An Overview" in *Managing Complex Networks: Strategies for the Public Sector*. W.J.M. Kickert, Eric-Hans Klijn and Joop F.M. Koppenjan (eds.). London, UK: Sage Publications, p. 35-61.

Kickert, Walter J.M., Erik-Hans Klijn and Joop F.M. Koppenjan (eds.). 1997. "Managing Networks in the Public Sector" in *Managing Complex Networks: Strategies for the Public Sector*. Walter J.M. Kickert, Erik-Hans Klijn and Joop F.M. Koppenjan (eds.). London, UK: Sage Publications, p. 166-191.

King, Cheryl Simrell, Kathryn M. Feltey and Bridget O'Neill Susel. 1998. "The Question of Participation in Public Administration," *Public Administration Review*, 58(4): 317-326.

Kingdon, John W. 2003. *Agendas, Alternatives, and Public Policies*. New York: Longman.

Kirby Report. 2003. See Senate Standing Committee on Social Affairs, Science and Technology.

Klijn, Erik-Hans. 1997. "Policy Networks: An Overview" in *Managing Complex Networks: Strategies for the Public Sector*. W.J.M. Kickert, Eric-Hans Klijn and Joop F.M. Koopenjan (eds.). London, UK: Sage Publications, p. 14-34.

Klijn, Erik-Hans and G. Teisman. 1997. "Strategies and Games in Networks" in *Managing Complex Networks: Strategies for the Public Sector*. W.J.M. Kickert, Eric-Hans Klijn, and Joop F.M. Koppenjan (eds.). London, UK: Sage Publications, p. 98-118.

Klijn, Erik-Hans, Joop F.M. Koppenjan, and Katrien Termeer. 1995. "Managing Networks in the Public Sector: A Theoretical Study of Management Strategies in Policy Networks," *Public Administration*, 73(autumn): 437-454.

Klitgaard, Robert and Gregory F. Treverton. 2004. "Assessing Partnerships: New Forms of Collaboration" in *Collaboration: Using Networks and Partnerships*. John M. Kamensky and Thomas J. Burlin (eds.). Lanham, MD: Rowman and Littlefield, p. 21-60.

Kooiman, Jan. 2000. "Societal Governance: Levels, Modes, and Orders of Social-Political Interaction" in *Debating Governance: Authority, Steering, and Democracy*. Jon Pierre (ed.). Oxford, UK: Oxford University Press, p. 138-164.

Koppenjan, Joop F.M. and Erik-Hans Klijn. 2004. *Managing Uncertainties in Networks*. London, UK and New York, NY: Routledge.

Laforest, Rachel and Michael Orsini. 2005. "Evidence-based Engagement in the Voluntary Sector: Lessons from Canada," *Social Policy and Administration*, 39(5): 481-97.

Lake, David A. and Wendy H. Wong. 2009. "The Politics of Networks: Interests, Power, and Human Rights Norms" in *Networked Politics: Agency, Power, and Governance*. Miles Kahler (ed.). Ithaca, NY and London, UK: Cornell University Press, p. 127-150.

Lalonde, Marc. 1974. *A New Perspective on the Health of Canadians*. Ottawa: Department of National Health and Welfare.

Lasker, Roz D., Elisa S. Weiss and Rebecca Miller. 2001. "Partnership Synergy: A Practical Framework for Studying and Strengthening the Collaborative Advantage," *The Millbank Quarterly*, 79(2): 179-205.

Last, J.M. 1998. *Health and Human Ecology*. 2nd ed. New York: McGraw-Hill Medical Publishing.

Laumann, Edward O. and David Knoke. 1987. *The Organizational State: Social Choice in National Policy Domains*. Madison, WI: University of Wisconsin Press.

Lazar, Harvey. 2006. "The Intergovernmental Dimensions of the Social Union: A Sectoral Analysis," *Canadian Public Administration*, 49(1): 23-45.

Lee, Kelley and Hilary Goodman. 2002. "Global Policy Networks: The Propagation of Health Care Financing Reform Since the 1980s" in *Health Policy in a Globalising World*. Kelley Lee, Kent Buse and Suzanne Fustukian (eds.) Cambridge, UK: Cambridge University Press, p. 97-119.

Lee, Kelley, Suzanne Fustukian, and Kent Buse. 2002. "An Introduction to Global Health Policy" in *Health Policy in a Globalising World*. Kelley Lee, Kent Buse and Suzanne Fustukian (eds.). Cambridge, UK: Cambridge University Press, p. 3-17.

Lencucha, Raphael, Ronald Labonté and Michael J. Rouse. 2010. "Beyond Idealism and Realism: Canadian NGO/Government Relations During the Negotiation of the FCTC," *Journal of Public Health Policy*, 31(1): 74-87.

Lindquist, Evert A. 1992. "Public Managers and Policy Communities: Learning to Meet New Challenges," *Canadian Public Administration*, 35(2): 127-159.

Lipnack, Jessica and Jeffrey Stamps. 1994. *The Age of the Network*. New York: John Wiley and Sons.

Lozon, Jeffrey C. and L. Miin Alikhan. 2007. "Canada's Public Health System: Is the Pace of Progress Sufficient," *Healthcare Papers*, 7(3): 52-59.

Luciani, Silvana and Neil J. Berman. 2000. "Status Report: Canadian Strategy for Cancer Control," *Chronic Diseases in Canada*, 21(1).

Macdonald, Théodore H. 2008. *Sacrificing the WHO to the Highest Bidder*. Oxford, UK or New York, NY: Radcliffe Publishing.

Magnusson, Roger S. 2007. "Non-communicable Diseases and Global Health Governance: Enhancing Global Processes to Improve Health Development," *Globalization and Health*, 3(2).

Mamudu, Hadaii. M. and S.A. Glantz. 2009. "Civil Society and the Negotiation of the Framework Agreement for Tobacco Control," *Global Public Health*, 4(2): 150-169.

Mamudu, Hadii M., Ross Hammond, and Stanton Glantz. 2008. "Tobacco Industry Attempts to Counter the World Bank Report *Curbing the Epidemic* and Obstruct the WHO Framework Convention on Tobacco Control," *Social Science and Medicine*, 67: 1690-1699.

Mandell, Myrna P. and Toddi A. Steelman. 2003. "Understanding What Can Be Accomplished Through Interorganizational Innovations: The Importance of Typologies, Context and Management Strategies," *Public Management Review*, 5(2): 197-224.

Margetts, Barrie. 2004. "Editorial," *Public Health Nutrition*, 7(3): 361-363.

Martin, (The Hon.) Paul Sr. 1948. "A National Health Program for Canada," *Canadian Journal of Public Health*, 39 (June): 219-226.

McCloskey, Michael. 2000. "Problems with Using Collaboration to Shape Environment Public Policy," *Valparaiso University Law Review*, 34: 423-434.

McKenna, Peter. 2009. "The Flu Fight Should Be Federal Territory," *Ottawa Citizen*, November 18.

McMillan, Alan and Seema Nagpal. 2007. "The Public Health System in Canada: Not Meeting the Needs of Canadians," *Healthcare Papers*, 7(3): 60-65.

McPherson, Charmaine M., Janice K. Popp and Ronald R. Lindstrom. 2007. "Re-examining the Paradox of Structure: A Child Health Network Perspective," *Healthcare Papers*, 7(2): 46-52.

Miller, Chris. 1998. "Canadian Non-Profits in Crisis: The Need for Reform," *Social Policy and Administration*, 32(4): 401-419.

Miller, Chris. 1999. "Tough Questions Avoided: The Broadbent Report on the Voluntary Sector," *Policy Options*, 20(8): 75.

Mingus, Matthew S. 2001. "From Subnet to Supranet: A Proposal for a Comparative Network Framework to Examine Network Interactions Across Borders" in *Getting Results Through Collaboration*. Myrna P. Mandell (ed.). Westport, CT: Quorum Books, p. 30-48.

Mintrom, Michael and Sandra Vergari. 1996. "Advocacy Coalitions, Policy Entrepreneurs, and Policy Change," *Policy Studies Journal*, 24(3): 420-434.

Mitchell, Shannon M. and Stephen M. Shortell. 2000. "The Governance and Management of Effective Community Health Partnerships: A Typology for Research, Policy, and Practice," *The Milbank Quarterly*, 78(2): 241-289.

Moore, Mark. H. 2009. "Networked Government: Survey of Rationales, Forms, and Techniques" in *Unlocking the Power of Networks: Keys to High-Performance Government*. Stephen Goldsmith and Donald F. Kettl (eds.). Washington, DC: Brookings University Press, p. 190-228.

Morison, John. 2000. "The Government-Voluntary Sector Compacts: Governance, Governmentality, and Civil Society," *Journal of Law and Society*, 27(1): 98-132.

Mowat, David and David Butler-Jones. 2007. "Public Health in Canada: A Difficult History," *Healthcare Papers*, 7(3): 31- 36.

Mowat, David and Dick de Jong. 2003. "Resource Document and Discussion Paper on Public Health." Unpublished paper. Ottawa: Population and Public Health Branch, Health Canada.

Moynihan, Donald P. 2005. *Leveraging Collaborative Networks in Infrequent Emergency Situations*. Washington, DC: IBM Center for the Business of Government.

Moynihan, Donald P. 2009. "The Network Governance of Crisis Response: Case Studies of Incident Command Systems," *Journal of Public Administration Research and Theory*, 19(4): 895-915.

National Advisory Committee on SARS and Public Health. 2003. *Learning from SARS (Naylor Report)*. Ottawa: Health Canada.

National Collaborating Centre for Healthy Public Policy. 2008. *Integrated Governance and Healthy Public Policy: Two Canadian Examples.* Unpublished paper.

Nelson, Lisa S. 2001. "Environmental Networks: Relying on Process or Outcome for Motivation" in *Getting Results through Collaboration.* Myrna P. Mandell (ed.). Westport, CT: Quorum Books, p. 89-102.

Naylor Report. 2003. See National Advisory Committee on SARS and Public Health.

Norum, Kaare R. 2005. "World Health Organization's Global Strategy on Diet, Physical Activity and Health: The Process Behind the Scenes," *Scandinavian Journal of Nutrition,* 49(2): 83-88.

O'Connell, Brian. 1996. "A Major Transfer of Government Responsibility to Voluntary Organizations? Proceed with Caution," *Public Administration Review,* 56(3): 222-225.

O'Leary, Rosemay. 2010. "Guerrilla Employees: Should Managers Nurture, Tolerate, or Terminate Them?" *Public Administration Review,* January/February: 8-19.

Oliver, Thomas R. 2006. "The Politics of Public Health Policy," *American Revue of Public Health,* 27: 195-233.

O'Neill, Michel, Vincent Lemieux, Gisèle Groleau, Jean-Paul Fortin and Paul A. Lamarche. 1997. "Coalition Theory as a Framework for Understanding and Implementing Intersectoral Health-Related Interventions," *Health Promotion International,* 12(1): 79-87.

Orbinski, James. 2007. "Global Health, Social Movements, and Governance" in *Governing Global Health: Challenge, Response, Innovation.* Andrew F. Cooper, John J. Kirton and Ted Schrecker (eds.). Burlington, VT: Ashgate, p. 29-40.

O'Toole, Laurence J. Jr. 1997. "Treating Networks Seriously: Practical and Research-based Agendas in Public Administration," *Public Administration Review,* 57(1): 45-52.

O'Toole, Laurence J. Jr. 2010. "The Ties That Bind? Networks, Public Administration, and Political Science," *PS: Political Science and Politics,* 43(1): 7-14.

O'Toole, Laurence J. Jr., K.I. Hanf and P.L. Hupe. 1997. "Managing Implementation Processes in Networks" in *Managing Complex Networks: Strategies for the Public Sector*. W.J.M. Kickert, Erik-Hans Klijn and Joop F.M. Koppenjan (eds.). London, UK: Sage Publications, p. 137-151.

Ottawa Charter for Health Promotion. 1986. Ottawa: World Health Organization; Health and Welfare Canada; Canadian Public Health Association.

Painter, Martin. 2001. "Multi-level Governance and the Emergence of Collaborative Federal Institutions in Australia," *Policy and Politics*, 29(2): 137-150.

Pan-Canadian Public Health Network. 2010a. *Public Health Network Operational Review Project: Final Report*. Ottawa: Public Health Agency of Canada.

Pan-Canadian Public Health Network. 2010b. *Public Health Network Operational Review Project: Final Report – Executive Summary*. Ottawa: Public Health Agency of Canada.

Pan-Canadian Public Health Network. 2010c. *Annual Report 2010-2011*. Ottawa: Public Health Agency of Canada.

Papadoupolis, Yannis. 2007. "Problems of Democratic Accountability in Network and Multilevel Governance," *European Law Journal*, 13(4): 469-486.

Paquet, Gilles. 2008. "Governance as Stewardship," *www.optimumonline*, 38(4): 14-46.

Paquet, Gilles. 2009a. *Crippling Epistemologies and Governance Failures: A Plea for Experimentalism*. Ottawa: University of Ottawa Press.

Paquet, Gilles. 2009b. *Scheming virtuously: the road to collaborative governance*. Ottawa: Invenire Books.

Paquet, Gilles. 2011. *Gouvernance collaborative : Un antimanuel*. Montreal: Liber.

Partners in Public Health. 2005. Final Report of the Federal/Provincial/Territorial Special Task Force on Public Health. Ottawa: Health Canada.

Petak, William J. 1985. "Emergency Management: A Challenge for Public Administration," *Public Administration Review*, (special issue): 3-7.

Peters, B. Guy. 1998. *Managing Horizontal Government: The Politics of Coordination*. Ottawa: Canadian Centre for Management Development, Research Paper no. 21.

Peters, B. Guy. 2007. "Virtuous and Viscous Circles in Democratic Network Governance" in *Theories of Democratic Network Governance*. Eva Sorenson and Jacob Torfing (eds.). New York: Palgrave Macmillan, p. 61-76.

Phillips, Susan D. 2001. "From Charity to Clarity: Reinventing Federal Government-Voluntary Sector Relationships," *The Philanthropist*, 16(4): 240-262.

Phillips, Susan D. 2004. "The Myths of Horizontal Governance: Is the Third Sector Really a Partner?" Paper presented to the International Society for Third-sector Research Conference, Toronto, ON.

Phillips, Susan D. and Karine Levasseur. 2004. "The Snakes and Ladders of Accountability: Contradictions between Contracting and Collaborating for Canada's Voluntary Sector," *Canadian Public Administration*, 47(4): 451-474.

Phillips, Susan D. and Katherine A. Graham. 2000. "Hand-in-Hand: When Accountability Meets Collaboration in the Voluntary Sector" in *The Nonprofit Sector in Canada: Roles and Relationships*. Keith G. Banting (ed.). Montreal and Kingston: McGill-Queen's University Press, p. 149-190.

Pierre, Jon (ed.). 2000. *Debating Governance*. Oxford, UK: Oxford University Press.

Pierre, Jon and B. Guy Peters (eds.). 2000. *Governance, Politics, and the State*. New York, NY: St. Martin's Press.

Pierre, Jon and B. Guy Peters. 2005. *Governing Complex Societies*. Hampshire, UK: Palgrave Macmillan.

Posner, Paul. 2002. "Accountability Challenges of Third-Party Government" in *The Tools of Government: A Guide to the New Government*. Lester M. Salamon (ed.). Oxford, UK: Oxford University Press, p. 523-564.

Posner, Paul. 2009. "Networks in the Shadow of Government: The Chesapeake Bay Program" in *Unlocking the Power of Networks: Keys to High-Performance Government*. Stephen Goldsmith and Donald F. Kettl (eds.). Washington, DC: Brookings University Press, p. 62-94.

Prevention of Violence Canada. 2009. *Working Together for a Canada Free of Violence*. Presentation to the Fifth Annual Town Hall Meeting.

Prince, Michael J. 2006. "A Cancer Control Strategy and Deliberative Federalism: Modernizing Health Care and Democratizing Intergovermental Relations," *Canadian Public Administration*, 49(4): 468-485.

Privy Council Office. 2001. *An Accord Between the Government of Canada and the Voluntary Sector*. Ottawa: Voluntary Sector Task Force, Privy Council Office.

Privy Council Office. 2011. *A Public Service for Challenging Times: Fifth Report of the Prime Minister's Advisory Committee on the Public Service*. Ottawa: Government of Canada.

Pross, A. Paul. *Group Politics and Public Policy*. 1986. Toronto, ON: Oxford University Press.

Provan, Keith G. and H. Brinton Milward. 2001. "Do Networks Really Work? A Framework for Evaluating Public-Sector Organizational Networks," *Public Management Review*, 61(4): 414-423.

Provan, Keith G. and Patrick Kenis. 2007. "Modes of Network Governance: Structure, Management, and Effectiveness," *Journal of Public Administration Research and Theory*, 18: 229-252.

Public Health Agency of Canada. *Health Goals for Canada*. www. phac-aspc.gc.ca/hgc-osc/home.html.

Public Health Agency of Canada Act. 2006. Ottawa: Government of Canada.

Public Health Agency of Canada. 2007. *Crossing Sectors – Experiences in Intersectoral Action, Public Policy and Health*. Ottawa: Public Health Agency of Canada.

Public Health Agency of Canada. 2008. *Report of the Chief Public Health Officer of Canada on the State of Public Health in Canada*. Ottawa: Public Health Agency of Canada.

Public Health Agency of Canada. 2010. *Lessons Learned Review: Public Health Agency of Canada and Health Canada Response to the 2009 H1N1 Pandemic*. Ottawa: Public Health Agency of Canada.

Rainey, Glenn W. Jr. and Terry Busson. 2001. "Assessing and Modeling Determinants of Capacity for Actors in Networked Public Programs" in *Getting Results Through Collaboration*. Myrna P. Mandell (ed.). Westport, CT: Quorum Books, p. 49-70.

Reinicke, Wolfgang H. 1999-2000. "The Other World Web: Global Public Policy Networks," *Foreign Policy*, (Winter): 44-57.

Reinicke, Wolfgang H. and Francis Deng. 2000. *Critical Choices: The United Nations, Networks, and the Future of Global governance*. Ottawa: International Development Research Centre.

Rhodes, R.A.W. 1997. *Understanding Governance: Reflexivity and Accountability*. Buckingham, UK: Open University Press.

Rhodes, R.A.W. 2000. "Governance and Public Administration" in *Debating Governance: Authority, Steering, and Democracy*. Jon Pierre (ed.). Oxford, UK: Oxford University Press, p. 54-90.

Rhodes, R.A.W. and John Wanna. 2007. "The Limits to Public Value, or Rescuing Responsible Government from the Platonic Guardians," *The Australian Journal of Public Administration*, 66(4): 406-421.

Riley, Barbara L. and Annamaria Feltracco. 2002. *Situational Analysis of the Canadian Heart Health Initiative: Final Report*. Unpublished document produced for Health Canada, Ottawa.

Riley, Barbara L., S. Martin Taylor and Susan J. Elliott. 2003. "Organizational Capacity and Implementation Change: A Comparative Case Study of Heart Health Promotion in Ontario Public Health Agencies," *Health Education Research*, 18(6): 754-769.

Riley, Barbara L., Sylvie Stachenko, Elinor Wilson, Dexter Harvey, Roy Cameron, Jane Farquharson, Catherine Donovan and Gregory Taylor. 2009. "Can the Canadian Heart Health Initiative Inform the Population Health Intervention Research Initiative for Canada?" *Canadian Journal of Public Health*, 100(1): 1-21.

Rittel, Horst W.J. and Melvin Webber. 1973. "Dilemmas in a General Theory of Planning," *Policy Sciences*, 4(2): 155-169.

Rocan, Claude. 2009. "Multi-level Collaborative Governance: The Canadian Heart Health Initiative," *www.optimumonline.ca*, 39(4): 1-16.

Rocan, Claude. 2010. "SARS, Public Health, and Network Governance," *www.optimumonline.ca*, 40(2): 61-77.

Roemer, Ruth, Allyn Taylor and Jean Larivière. 2005. "Origins of the WHO Framework Convention on Tobacco Control," *American Journal of Public Health*, 95(6): 936-938.

Romanow, Roy J. 2002. *Building on Values: The Future of Health Care in Canada – Final Report*. Commission on the Future of Health Care in Canada. Ottawa: Government of Canada.

Rosenau, James N. 2005. "Governance in the Twenty-First Century" in *The Global Governance Reader*. Rorden Wilkinson (ed.). London and New York: Routledge, p. 45-67.

Roussos, Stergios Tsai and Stephen B. Fawcett. 2000. "A Review of Collaborative Partnerships as a Strategy for Improving Community Health," *Annual Review of Public Health*, 21: 369-402.

Rutty, Christopher and Sue C. Sullivan. 2010. *This is Public Health: A Canadian History*. Ottawa: Canadian Public Health Association.

Sabatier, Paul A. 1988. "An Advocacy Coalition Framework of Policy Change and the Role of Policy-oriented Learning Therein," *Policy Sciences*, 21: 129-168.

Sabatier, Paul A. and Hank C. Jenkins-Smith. 1999. "The Advocacy Coalition Framework: An Assessment" in *Theories of the Policy Process*. Paul A. Sabatier (ed.). Boulder, CO: Westview Press, p. 117-167.

Salamon, Lester M. 1995. *Partners in Public Service: Government-Nonprofit Relations in the Modern Welfare State*. Baltimore and London: The John Hopkins University Press.

Salamon, Lester M. 1999. "Government-Nonprofit Relations in International Perspective" in *Nonprofits & Governments: Collaboration and Conflict*. Elizabeth T. Boris and Eugene Steuerle (eds.). Washington, DC: The Urban Institute Press, p. 329-367.

Salamon, Lester M. 2002. "The New Governance and the Tools of Public Action: An Introduction" in *The Tools of Government: A Guide to the New Government.* L.M. Salamon (ed.). Oxford, UK: Oxford University Press, p. 1-47.

Salamon, Lester M., S. Wojciech Sokolowski and Regina List. 1999. "Global Civil Society: An Overview" in *Global Civil Society: Dimensions of the Nonprofit Sector.* vol. 2. Salamon, Sokolowski, and Associates (eds.). Bloomfield, CT: Kumarian Press, p. 3-60.

Salamon, Lester M., S. Wojciech Sokolowski and Regina List. 2003. *Global Civil Society: An Overview.* Baltimore, MD.: John Hopkins University.

SARS Commission. 2004. *Interim Report: SARS and Public Health in Ontario (Campbell Report).* Toronto: Government of Ontario.

SARS Commission. 2005a. *Second Interim Report: SARS and Public Health Legislation (Campbell Report).* Toronto: Government of Ontario.

SARS Commission. 2005b. *Final Report (Campbell Report).* Toronto: Government of Ontario.

Schaap, L. and M.J.W. van Twist. 1997. "The Dynamics of Closedness in Networks" in *Managing Complex Networks: Strategies for the Public Sector.* W.J.M. Kickert, Eric-Hans Klijn and Joop F.M. Koppenjan (eds.). London, UK: Sage Publications, p. 62-78.

Scharf, F.W. 1994. "Games Real Actors Could Play: Positive and Negative Coordination in Embedded Negotiations," *Journal of Theoretical Politics,* 6(1): 27-53.

Schlager, Edella. 1995. "Policy Making and Collective Action: Defining Coalitions within the Advocacy Coalition Framework," *Policy Sciences,* 28(3): 243-270.

Scholte, Jan Aart. 2005. "Civil Society and Democracy in Global Governance" in *The Global Governance Reader.* Rorden Wilkinson (ed.). London and New York: Routledge.

Senate Standing Committee on Social Affairs, Science and Technology. 2002. *The Health of Canadians – The Federal Role.* Ottawa: Senate of Canada.

Senate Standing Committee on Social Affairs, Science and Technology. 2003. *Reforming Health Protection and Promotion in Canada: Time to Act (Kirby Report.)* Ottawa: Senate of Canada.

Senate Standing Committee on Social Affairs, Science and Technology. 2006. *Out of the Shadows at Last: Transforming Mental Health, Mental Illness and Addiction Services in Canada.* Ottawa: Senate of Canada.

Simmons, Julie M. 2008. "Democratizing Executive Federalism: The Role of Non-Governmental Actors in Intergovernmental Agreements" in *Canadian Federalism: Performance, Effectiveness, and Legitimacy.* Second Edition. Herman Bakvis and Grace Skogstad (eds.). Oxford, UK: Oxford University Press, p. 355-379.

Slaughter, Anne-Marie. 2004. *A New World Order.* Princeton, NJ: Princeton University Press.

Sorensen, Eva. 2002. "Democratic Theory and Network Governance," *Administrative Theory & Praxis,* 24(4): 693-720.

Sorensen, Eva. 2006. "Metagovernance: The Changing Role of Politicians in Processes of Democratic Governance," *American Review of Public Administration,* 36(1): 98-114.

Sorensen, Eva and Jacob Torfing. 2007. "Theoretical Approaches to Governance Network Failure" in *Theories of Democratic Network Governance.* Eva Sorensen and Jacob Torfing (eds.). Hampshire, UK: Palgrave Macmillan, p. 95-110.

Sorensen, Eva and Jacob Torfing. 2009. "Making Governance Networks Effective and Democratic Through Meta-governance," *Public Administration,* 87(2): 234-58.

Stachenko, Sylvie. 2001. "Case Study: the Canadian Heart Health Initiative" in *Evaluation in Health Promotion.* Irving Rootman, Michael Goodstadt, Brian Hyndman, David V. McQueen, Louise Potvin, Jane Springett and Erio Ziglio (eds.). Copenhagen: WHO Regional Publications, European Series, no. 92, p. 463-473.

Stoker, Gerry. 1995. "Regime Theory and Urban Politics" in *Theories of Urban Politics.* D. Judge, G. Stoker and H. Wolman (eds.). London, UK: Sage Publications, p. 54-71.

Stoker, Gerry. 1998. "Governance as Theory: Five Propositions." *UNESCO, ISSJ* 155/1998, p. 17-28.

Stoker, Gerry. 2006. "Public Value Management: A New Narrative for Networked Governance?" *American Review of Public Administration,* 36(1): 41-57.

Takahashi, Lois and Gail Smutny. 2002. "Collaborative Windows and Organizational Governance: Exploring the Formation and Demise of Social Service Partnerships," *Non-Profit and Voluntary Sector Quarterly,* 31(2):165-185.

Tam, Theresa, Jill Sciberras, Beatrice Mullington and Arlene King. 2005. "Fortune Favours the Prepared Mind," *Canadian Journal of Public Health,* 96(6): 406-408.

Taylor, Allyn. 2002. "Global Governance, International Health Law and WHO: Looking Towards the Future," *Bulletin of the World Health Organization,* 80(12): 975-980.

Taylor, Marilyn. 1997. *The Best of Both Worlds: The Voluntary Sector and Local Government.* York, UK: Joseph Rowntree Foundation.

Termeer, C.J.A.M. and Joop F.M. Koppenjan. 1997. "Managing Perceptions in Networks" in *Managing Complex Networks: Strategies for the Public Sector.* W.J.M. Kickert, Eric-Hans Klijn and Joop F.M. Koppenjan (eds.) London, UK: Sage Publications, p. 79-97.

Teisman, Geert R. and Erik-Hans Klijn. 2002. "Partnership Arrangements: Governmental Rhetoric or Governance Scheme?" *Public Administration Review,* 62(2): 197-205.

Thatcher, Mark. 1998. "The Development of Policy Network Analyses: From Modest Origins to Overarching Frameworks," *Journal of Theoretical Politics,* 10(4): 389-416.

Tierney, Kathleen J. 1985. "Emergency Medical Preparedness and Response in Disasters: The Need for Interorganizational Coordination," *Public Administration Review,* special issue.

Tilson, Hugh and Bobbie Berkowitz. 2006. "The Public Health Enterprise: Examining our Twenty-First-Century Policy Challenges," *Health Affairs,* 25(4): 900-910.

Tsasis, Peter. 2008. "The Politics of Governance: Government-Voluntary Sector Relationships," *Canadian Public Administration,* 51(2): 265-290.

Tukuitonga, Colin and Ingrid Keller. 2005. "Implementing the World Health Organization Global Strategy on Diet, Physical Activity and Health," *Scandinavian Journal of Nutrition,* 49(3): 122-126.

Turnock, Bernard J. and Christopher Atchison. 2002. "Governmental Public Health in the United States: The Implications of Federalism," *Health Affairs,* 21(6): 68-78.

United Kingdom/Compact Voice/Commission for the Compact/ Local Government Association. 1998. *The Compact on Relations between Government and The Third Sector in England.* London and Birmingham: Crown copyright.

Vangen, Siv and Chris Huxham. 2003. "Nurturing Collaborative Relations: Building Trust in Interorganizational Collaboration," *The Journal of Applied Behavioral Science,* 39(1): 5-31.

Van Kersbergen, Kees and Frans Van Waarden. 2004. "'Governance' as a Bridge Between Disciplines: Cross-disciplinary Inspiration Regarding Shifts in Governance and Problems of Governability, Accountability and Legitimacy," *European Journal of Political Research,* 43: 143-171.

Voluntary Sector Initiative Impact Evaluation: Lessons Learned from the Voluntary Sector Initiative (2000-2005). 2009. Final Report. Ottawa: Human Resources and Skills Development Canada.

Waddell, Steve and L. David Brown. 1997. "Fostering Intersectoral Partnering: A Guide to Promoting Cooperation Among Government, Business, and Civil Society Actors," *IDR Reports,* 13(3): 1-26.

Wagenaar, Hendrik and S.D. Noam Cook. 2003. "Understanding Policy Practices: Action, Dialectic, and Deliberation in Policy Analysis" in *Deliberative Policy Analysis: Understanding Governance in the Network Society.* Maarten A. Hajer and Hendrick Wagenaar (eds.). Cambridge, UK: Cambridge University Press, p. 139-171.

Walker Report. 2004. See Expert Panel on SARS and Infectious Disease Control.

Wallace, W. Stewart (ed.). 1948. "Public Health in Canada." *The Encyclopedia of Canada*. vol. V. Toronto: University Associates of Canada.

Walt, Gill and Lucy Gilson. 1994. "Reforming the Health Sector in Developing Countries: The Central Role of Analysis," *Health Policy and Planning*, 9(4): 353-370.

Waugh, William L. Jr. and Gregory Streib. 2006. "Collaboration and Leadership for Effective Emergency Management," *Public Administration Review*, December special issue.

Waxman, Amalia. 2005. "Why a Global Strategy on Diet, Physical Activity and Health?" *World Review on Nutrition and Diet*, 95: 162-166.

Webster, Paul. 2009. "Aboriginal Groups Seek Representation on Pan-Canadian Public Health Network," *Canadian Medical Association Journal*, 181(11): 781-782.

Weiss, Thomas G. 2005. "Governance, Good Governance and Global Governance: Conceptual and Actual Challenges" in *The Global Governance Reader*. Rorden Wilkinson (ed.). London and New York: Routledge, p. 69-88.

Wenger, E.C. and W.M. Snyder. 2000. "Communities of Practice: The Organizational Frontier," *Harvard Business Review*, (Jan-Feb): 139-145.

Wilkenfeld, Judith P. 2005. "Saving the World from Big Tobacco: The Real Coalition of the Willing." Working Paper from the Ridgway Working Group on Challenges to U.S. Foreign and Military Policy. Pittsburgh: Ridgway Center, University of Pittsburgh.

Wilson, Christopher. 2011. "On Collaboration," *www.optimumonline.ca*, 41(1): 15-31.

Wilson, Kumanan. 2004. "The Complexities of Multi-level Governance in Public Health," *Canadian Journal of Public Health*, 95(6): 409-12.

Wilson, Kumanan. 2006. "Pandemic Threats and the Need for New Emergency Public Health Legislation in Canada," *Healthcare Policy*, 2(2): 35-42.

Wilson, Kumanan, Barbara von Tigerstrom and Christopher McDougall. 2008. "Protecting Global Health Security Through the International Health Regulations: Requirements and Challenges," *Canadian Medical Association Journal*, 179(1): 44-48.

Wilson, Kumanan and Harvey Lazar. 2005. "Planning for the Next Pandemic Threat: Defining the Federal Role in Public Health Emergencies," *IRPP Policy Matters*, 6(5): 1-36.

Wilson, Kumanan and Harvey Lazar. 2008. "Creative Federalism and Public Health" in *Special Series: The Role of Federalism in Protecting the Public's Health*. Kingston, ON: Institute of Intergovernmental Relations, Queen's University.

Witte, Jan Martin, Charlotte Streck and Thorsten Benner. 2003. "The Road from Johannesburg: What Future for Partnerships in Global Environmental Governance?" in *Peril or Progress? Partnerships and Networks in Global Environmental Governance. The Post-Jahannesburg Agenda*. Jan Martin Witte, Charlotte Streck and Thorsten Benner (eds.). Washington, DC: Global Public Policy Institute, p. 59-84.

World Health Organization. 2003a. *Process for a Global Strategy on Diet, Physical Activity and Health*. Geneva: World Health Organization.

World Health Organization. 2003b. *World Health Report*. Geneva: World Health Organization.

World Health Organization. 2008a. *Closing the Gap in a Generation: Health Equity Through Action on the Social Determinants of Health*. Geneva: World Health Organization.

World Health Organization. 2008b. *Health Equity Through Intersectoral Action: An Analysis of 18 Country Case Studies*. Geneva: World Health Organization.

World Health Organization. 2009. *History of the WHO Framework Convention on Tobacco Control*. Geneva: World Health Organization.

Young, Dennis R. 1999. "Complementary, Supplementary, or Adversarial? A Theoretical and Historical Examination of Nonprofit-Government Relations in the United States" in *Nonprofits and Government: Collaboration and Conflict*. Elizabeth T. Boris and C. Eugene Steuerle (eds.). Washington, DC: The Urban Institute Press, p. 37-79.

Young, Dennis R. 2000. "Alternative Models of Government-Non-profit Sector Relations," *Non-profit and Voluntary Sector Quarterly*, 29(1): 149-172.

Other titles published by INVENIRE

Titles in the Collaborative Decentred Metagovernance Series

www.ingramcontent.com/pod-product-compliance
Lightning Source LLC
Chambersburg PA
CBHW071736270326
41928CB00013B/2700